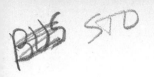
ngevity

**DO NOT REMOVE
CARDS FROM POCKET**

**ALLEN COUNTY PUBLIC LIBRARY
FORT WAYNE, INDIANA 46802**

You may return this book to any agency, branch,
or bookmobile of the Allen County Public Library.

DEMCO

Lifestyle for Longevity

Norman Ford

Para Research
Gloucester
Massachusetts

Lifestyle for Longevity
by Norman Ford

Library of Congress Card Number: 82-62228
International Standard Book Number: 0-914918-63-X

Printed by Alpine Press, Inc.
on 55-pound Surtone II Antique
Edited by Marah Ren and Emily McKeigue
Cover Design by Ralph Poness
Typeset by Patrice LeBlanc

Published by Para Research, Inc.
85 Eastern Ave.
Gloucester, Massachusetts 01930

Manufactured in the United States of America

First Printing October 1984, 3,000 copies

Acknowledgments

In developing the life extension program in this book, I have drawn on the work of many researchers in the science of life extension. Most of the data in this book are derived from controlled studies, many funded by the United States government and carried out by scientists and gerontologists associated with leading universities and university medical centers.

Other data were researched from studies reported in professional journals, and from the verified results of studies and investigations conducted in government- or university-sponsored programs. I have also drawn on my own computerized analysis of the lifestyle profiles of two hundred American centenarians.

So many direct and indirect sources were consulted in researching this book that it is impractical to acknowledge every one. However, I would like to acknowledge my debt to the work of: Dr. Julius Axelrod, National Institutes of Health; Vern L. Bengston, Ph.D., Andrus Gerontology Center, University of Southern California; Johan Bjorksten, Bjorksten Research Foundation, Madison, Wisconsin; Dr. Henry Blackburn, University of Minnesota; Dr. Walter Bortz, Stanford University Medical School; Lester Breslow, Ph.D., School of Public Health, University of California, Los Angeles; Dr. William P. Castelli, medical director, Framingham Heart Study; W. Donner Denckla M.D., Roche Institute of Molecular Biology; Herbert DeVries, Ph.D., Andrus Gerontology Center, University of Southern California; Dr. Hans Fisher, Department of Nutrition, Rutgers University; Dr. Philip Gold and Dr. Frederick K. Goodwin, National Institutes of Mental Health; Joseph S. Goldstein and Dr. Scott Grundy, University of Texas Science Center, Dallas; Robert Good, M.D., Memorial Sloan-Kettering Cancer Center, New York;

Denham Harman, M.D., University of Nebraska Medical Center; Ronald L. Harper, Ph.D., director, Gerontology Center, University of Kansas; Raymond Harris, M.D., Center for the Study of Aging, Albany, New York; Fred Mattson, Ph.D., University of California School of Medicine, San Diego; Donna Maxwell, National Institutes on Aging, Bethesda, Maryland; Hamish Munro, M.D., Human Nutrition Research Center on Aging, United States Department of Agriculture, Boston; Iris Fletcher Norstrand, M.D., director, Neuro-Chemistry Laboratory, VA Medical Center, Brooklyn; Dr. Erdman Palmore, Center for the Study of Aging and Human Development, Duke University; Leon Pastalan, Ph.D., Institute of Gerontology, University of Michigan; Nathan Pritikin, Longevity Center, Santa Monica, California; Dr. Paul Rosch, director, American Institute of Stress, Yonkers, New York; Dr. Edward L. Schneider, Gerontology Research Center, National Institutes on Aging, Baltimore; Hans Selye, Institute of Experimental Medicine and Surgery, University of Montreal; Patricia A. Wagner, Ph.D., University of Florida, Gainesville; Roy L. Walford, Ph.D., Department of Pathology, UCLA Medical Center; Dr. Harold Ward, Director, Stress Medicine Laboratory, University of California, San Diego; John Yudkin, Department of Nutrition, London University, London, England.

I would also like to acknowledge these institutions, which supplied copies of studies and a wealth of scientific information that I used in researching this book: American Longevity Association, Torrance, California; Arthur Vining Davis Center for Behavioral Neurology, San Diego; Center for Disease Control, Atlanta; Gerontology Center, Georgia State University, Atlanta; Research Services, Mayo Clinic, Rochester, Minnesota; Normative Aging Study, Veterans Administration, Boston; Institute of Gerontology, USSR Academy of Medical Sciences, Kiev, Ukraine; National Institutes on Aging-National Institutes of Health-Baltimore Longitudinal Study of the National Institutes on Aging, all divisions of the United States Department of Health and Human Services.

Contents

Lifex Constants

Introduction

This book is designed to show how you can extend the number of active, productive, healthful years *in the middle of your life.*

Instead of these middle years lasting from ages 35 to 60, you will learn how you can make them stretch longer, perhaps even from ages 35 to 85. If you are already over 60, and approaching what most of us currently consider to be old age, you will learn how you can become functionally younger. You may well be able to re-enter your middle years again and extend them by as much as a decade.

You can achieve this by incorporating into your lifestyle certain traits and habits that scientists have found occur in the lifestyle profiles of many long-lived people throughout the world. These life extension constants, called Lifex Constants in this book, form the basis of the life extension program described in these pages.

The main thrust of life extension research is taking place on two levels: first, the biochemical approach, which views life extension in terms of a mechanistic body composed of billions of cells; and second, the lifestyle approach, which views life extension in terms of a body mechanism whose well-being is governed by our personality traits and lifestyle habits.

As scientists have attempted to find cures for such diseases as cancer, heart disease and diabetes, an explosion of new information has emerged from every branch of biochemistry. Although few of these discoveries is likely to actually extend life, the concept of genetic engineering and similar biochemical techniques has captured the public's imagination. Many firmly believe that within a few years, biochemistry will produce a pill or hormone that will enable us to extend our lives by one or two decades or more.

While the media has heralded each biochemical discovery with a fanfare of publicity, the emerging results of hundreds of other studies that are concerned with life extension have been largely overlooked by all but a few professional gerontologists. These studies, from such widely divergent sources as stress management, gerontology, sociology, psychology, nutrition and physiotherapy, reveal that many of the factors that determine our life expectancy arise from our personality traits and lifestyle habits, while biochemistry plays a relatively minor role. The studies show that while we die of physical diseases that take place at the biochemical level, the underlying cause of these diseases is largely psychological.

We are dying of physical diseases that are psychological in origin. Cancer, for example, may be caused biochemically by a carcinogen; however, cancer can manifest only when the immune system is suppressed. The prime cause of immuno-suppression is unresolved emotional stress. Likewise, cholesterol deposits resulting from a diet high in fat work at the biochemical level to clog the arteries that supply blood to the heart. Surveys show that a large proportion of heart attacks are actually triggered when muscles enclosing the arteries constrict due to emotional pressure and stress.

In most cases, we are shortening our lives not because of biochemical factors in our cells but because of our emotional response to what is going on in our lives. We can begin to extend our lives by eliminating the personality and lifestyle risk factors that are currently causing us to die prematurely. We can replace them with health-building habits that can lengthen life.

One reason why this information has not been widely publicized is that much of the knowledge about life extension tends to be fragmented. Biochemists, for example, often know little of the parallel research being done by lifestyle investigators, and vice versa.

Rather than following a holistic trend, which centralizes and coordinates all information, the trend in life extension is toward increasing fragmentation. This is partly because studies are based on a single variable. For instance, a study may investigate the relationship of exercise to heart disease, but it is not in the nature of the scientific method to investigate the overall effects of both diet and exercise together on heart disease, or of exercise, diet and stress management combined on heart disease, cancer and diabetes.

Exemplifying this trend toward divergence is the existence of a dozen or more nationwide organizations and societies, each dedicated to finding a cure for a single disease. Thus we have groups such as the American Cancer Society, the National Cancer Institute, the American Heart Association, and the Framingham Heart Study, each concerned with investigating a single disease.

Some of these organizations—as well as individual scientists—have published details of diet and lifestyle habits designed to help prevent, or even to help reverse, the disease in which they specialize. As I compared the diets designed to prevent heart disease with others designed to prevent cancer, diabetes and other chronic diseases, I found that all of the diets were extraordinarily similar. The same applied to most other disease-prevention measures. They, too, were alike.

I also found that the same diet and lifestyle habits recommended to prevent these diseases were almost identical with the diet and lifestyle habits that occur in the profiles of most healthful, long-lived people.

My task in writing this book has been to integrate all of the scattered information into one unified theory of aging. As a result, this book accomplishes several things. First, it describes significant factors known to benefit health and life extension. Second, it outlines a program through which you can use a holistic approach to extend your life. Third, because life extension and improved health are synonymous, by following the program you will inevitably begin to experience a significantly improved level of health. Fourth, as I investigated the results of hundreds of studies from every branch of medicine, gerontology, and biochemistry, it became increasingly apparent that science already knows how to extend life.

What we have discovered is that people who live long and healthful lives are a special breed. Investigations show that they are confident, self-actualized people who are in full control of their health. Almost without exception, every person who has lived past ninety in fit and healthy condition has consciously or unconsciously been practicing the holistic approach to health and well-being.

The holistic methods they use consist of the same twenty-seven Lifex Constants that form the self-help program described in this book. Through incorporating the Constants into your lifestyle, you can transform your way of living so that you become one of that special breed of people who live a long and healthful life.

Norman D. Ford
Boulder, Colorado

1

Unlocking the Secrets
of Life Extension

At gerontology centers in America's most prestigious universities, scientists are making exciting discoveries about how we can live longer and healthier lives. By confining their studies only to fit, healthy people, researchers have developed a new model of aging.

Both Russian and American gerontologists now agree that the upper limit of human life is approximately 117 years and any claim to be older is probably exaggerated. Within this framework, gerontologists believe most of us could choose to live healthfully for 80 percent of the maximum lifespan—that is, until age 93 for men and 100 for women. Instead of our active, productive middle years lasting only from ages 35 to 60, studies show that in fit, healthy people, these middle years can stretch from ages 35 to 85. According to new aging models, we need not deteriorate much between ages 25 and 70, and we can remain healthy and vigorous until our late 80s and perhaps beyond.

What we now consider old age can be a time of activity and vigorous growth. Good health can last almost until the final day of life.

All this, gerontologists are learning, could be accomplished by incorporating into our lifestyle a series of health-building habits. These life extension constants—called "Lifex Constants" throughout this book—fall into two classes. The primarily *physical* constants include such health-enhancing factors as avoiding overeating; maintaining body weight at a desirable level; eating a low-fat, high-fiber diet; exercising briskly for an hour or more each day; and abstaining from smoking and stimulants and drugs including caffeine.

The primarily *psycho-social* constants include: responding to stress in a non-destructive way; staying mentally active; working hard throughout life at a fulfilling occupation; maintaining close ties with friends and family and avoiding living alone; having an active sex and love life; and having faith in something greater than ourselves.

Understandably, no single Lifex Constant will make us long-lived. Physical, social and psychological health risks are so interwoven that feeling (psychologically) worried or unloved about some (social) event in our lives can send us heading for the refrigerator to (physically) overeat. Studies have also demonstrated that negative emotions like resentment or fear can raise our cholesterol level and suppress the immune system, thereby lowering the body's defenses against infection.

Life Extension and Wellness Are the Same

The law of life extension is that whatever we do to improve our health today will extend our life in the future. Whatever we do to extend our life in future will improve our wellness today. Thus, life extension and wellness are synonymous. Through incorporating the Lifex Constants into your lifestyle, your health will begin to steadily improve, thereby improving the quality, as well as the quantity, of the extra years you will live.

Dr. William Esser, who runs a health ranch at Lake Worth, Florida, where many Lifex Constants are part of the daily routine, remarked to me that after a few weeks of practicing these life-sustaining habits, many guests begin to look and feel appreciably better. Surplus pounds melt away and joint stiffness disappears. Middle-aged fatigue and poor memory is replaced by youthful vigor and alertness. The eyes begin to sparkle and the hair takes on a new gloss. The back becomes straighter. The tummy flattens. With a new spring in his or her step, the chronologically 55-year-old begins to look, feel and function like a person who is, perhaps, biologically only 35.

This, then, is a book both about life extension and about how to presently enjoy exceptional health. By following the program, you eliminate the health risks that make people prematurely old, and you replace them with Lifex Constants that enhance your youthfulness.

The Lifex Constants include the same techniques used at life extension clinics around the world to control and inhibit such degenerative diseases as hypertension, heart disease, diabetes, rheumatoid arthritis, obesity and diverticulosis. Thousands of Americans, faced with financially-crippling cardiac surgery, have opted instead to enroll at cardiac rehabilitation centers where, under medical supervision, and with the aid of a few key Lifex Constants, they have managed to control their heart disease without resorting to either surgery or drugs.

How Soon Can Technology Overcome Aging?

Aging research only began in the 1950s with formation of such organizations as the International Association of Gerontology, the Soviet Institute of Gerontology, England's Nuffield Foundation, Switzerland's Institute of Experimental Gerontology and the United States' National Institutes of Health. Through these institutions, in an attempt to trace and find the cause of cancer, heart disease, diabetes and other diseases, vast and expensive epidemiological studies are under way to investigate exciting new frontiers in such fields as immunology, endocrine and neural mechanisms, protein synthesis and free radical pathology.

During the past decade, an explosion of new information has emerged from these and other studies. Hundreds of geneticists, molecular biologists, immunologists and nutritionists have made important discoveries which reveal how the body functions and how we age. Using modern technology, scientists have synthesized various "youth" and growth hormones that may eventually aid in prolonging life. Researchers have developed specific antibodies for a wide range of infectious diseases. To a limited extent, we have learned how to intervene in our body chemistry by using nutritional supplements.

These exciting new developments have caught the imagination of the public and have triggered an avalanche of media reports, magazine articles and books that focus on the biochemical approach to life extension. Discoveries have been dramatized and exaggerated to create the impression that an anti-aging pill is just a few years away.

In reality, however, the technology needed to extend life has yet to be developed. Advances in immunology and gene manipulation may eventually make it possible to slow the aging process; however, actual production of an anti-aging pill, drug or supplement—assuming one is ever discovered— could be decades away. Moreover, nothing is ever said about the adverse side effects and complications that are inherent in the use of many pharmaceuticals. Because excretion functions are slower in older people, the side effects of any drug intended to extend life are likely to offset the benefits. Even if a "youth" drug were discovered, production could be delayed for years by the FDA while the cost of the drug could prove financially out of reach of most people.

As a result, few gerontologists seriously believe that any existing form of biochemical or medical intervention will lead to a longevity revolution. This was confirmed in an interview with Dr. Edward Schneider of the National Institutes of Aging in the *Washington Post* of June 23, 1983. In response to a query about the possibility of an anti-aging pill, Dr. Schneider pointed out that "research into the nature of the aging process is a very exciting and promising area. But it's very new. We don't have the answers. All the evidence points to aging being caused by many, many factors. So to think that a single magic bullet, or a single anti-oxidant, can cure aging is extraordinarily naive."

Lifestyle Changes That Extend Life

Breakthroughs are indeed being made in life extension. But when it comes to finding life extension techniques that actually work, a curious thing is happening. Studies that cost billions to fund are unable to find solutions through any form of biochemical intervention. Instead of finding the answers in modern technology or in medical treatment or pharmaceuticals, researchers are being led right back to confirming the role of various health-promoting habits that have long been known to improve health and extend life.

After spending thirty years and untold billions of dollars in a search to cure cancer through drugs and technology, for example, the National Cancer Institute is now conducting an extensive longitudinal study on the anti-cancer properties of eating raw carrots. Meanwhile, the American Cancer Society is making a similar epidemiological study to discover which lifestyle habits and vitamin deficiencies increase cancer risk.

As scientists probe for the real causes of aging, they are finding increasingly persuasive evidence that although we die from a biochemical reaction like heart disease or cancer, the *cause* of these diseases lies in our psychological reaction to the social, occupational and economic influences in our lives.

Health and Long Life Are Psychological in Origin

Thus, the new thrust in gerontology research is the realization that 90 percent of the population die of physical dysfunctions that are psychological in origin. Even when an illness appears due to a physical cause like cholesterol deposits in the arteries, or overindulgence in food, alcohol or nicotine, the motivation that led to these physical conditions is psychological in origin.

Every year, for example, several hundred thousand Americans die of sudden cardiac death. Some 27 percent of these heart attacks have been found to occur in people who have nothing wrong with their heart or arteries. Yet closer analysis has revealed that these unexplained attacks frequently occur within twenty-four hours of a disturbing life event that leads to severe emotional stress.

The same rationale that led gerontologists to conclude that many causes of death are psychological in origin has also led to the counter-conclusion that almost all health and long life must also be psychological in origin. When we respond to a life situation with negative emotions such as anger or fear, our mind and body transform these inappropriate responses into suppression of the immune system, thereby reducing our resistance to infections and cancer.

Powerful emotional and psychological factors are the key to health and long life. It is how we view what is going on in our lives that determines our health and how long we will live. Understandably, since such inner forces are difficult to isolate and quantify, even by psychologists, they have largely been ignored in favor of physical and measurable biochemical factors.

Nonetheless, many surveys of life extension causes have concluded that physical habits and psycho-social lifestyle influences are far more dependable predictors of health and long life than any biochemical variables.

What Can We Expect from Life Extension Technology?

The biochemical approach to life extension begins at the cellular level and, hopefully, provides us with a body that works. Put another way, biochemical intervention seeks to provide us with an efficient vehicle, the body, for the journey through life. Through nutritional supplements, for example, it can supply more neurotransmitters to boost the function of neural pathways in the brain; or it can provide us with anti-oxidants that prevent free radical damage to our cells.

But we need more than a biochemically-efficient vehicle for the journey through life. We need a driver who can steer us successfully through all of life's adversities. The driver, of course, is the mind. Our success in attaining a healthful old age is determined more by our personality and lifestyle than by our cells.

Science Already Knows How to Extend Life

The fact that Lifex Constants are practical answers to life extension is borne out by such prominent gerontologists as Kenneth R. Pelletier, Ph.D., of the University of California School of Medicine. In his book *Longevity: Fulfilling Our Biological Heritage* (Delacorte, 1981), Pelletier writes that "despite the sophistication of genetic, biochemical and neuroendocrine research, the single, most accurate predictor of longevity is lifestyle."

Many gerontologists, in fact, agree that by incorporating the Lifex Constants into our personalities and living patterns, we can extend our lives. The personality and lifestyle factors that extend life and prolong youth have been scientifically documented. Countless cross-cultural studies of longevous people have identified lifestyle factors that make people live longer.

Misconceptions That Shorten Our Lives

If we already know how to enjoy good health and long life, why do not more of us adopt the Lifex Constants? Why do we see so few fit and healthy people in their 80s and 90s?

Much of the answer lies in popular misconceptions about aging. We see so many older people who have failed to make the Constants a part of their lives and who, as a result, are now feeble, that we assume sickness is the norm in the process of aging. A Louis Harris poll conducted for the National Council on Aging in the mid 1970s found that half of all adults expected poor health to be a problem in the later years.

Any vital, older person is considered exceptional. "My aunt Beatrice is ninety-one, walks five miles daily, stands tall and erect, and has a mind as clear as a bell."

In sharp contrast, according to new models of aging, life extension researchers now consider it normal for a woman to be physically fit and mentally active at 91. Conversely, some consider it abnormal for people to die of degenerative diseases in their 60s and 70s.

Several recent surveys have confirmed that as Americans enter the later years with increasing resources of health, education and income, life continues to improve. As we learn that through nutrition, exercise and other Lifex Constants we can retain our youthful vigor and agility, hundreds of older Americans are serving around the world in the Peace Corps. Thousands of others engage in competitive sports or enjoy long bicycle tours. Still others are assuming dynamic new roles in politics and other causes.

In fact, the annals are filled with records of people who made major contributions after reaching what we consider advanced ages. Grandma Moses was still painting at age 100 and so was Harry Lieberman; Bertrand Russell led peace drives at 94; Bernard Shaw wrote *Farfetched Fables* at 93; Eamon de Valera was president of Ireland at 91 and at the same age, Adolph Zukor was chairman of Paramount Pictures. Virtually all of these active people found that as they grew older, life became increasingly satisfying and rewarding.

Life Gets Better As We Age

Even the fittest older people slowly accumulate chronic conditions. Gradually, we lose our sense of taste and smell and most body responses eventually slow. But these seldom prevent fit and healthy older people from enjoying life.

The new models of aging have created a context in which the age of 65 is now considered the prime of life. If it is not, it is an indication that a person has failed to observe the Lifex Constants.

Most of the profiles on two hundred fit and healthy long-lived people in our files show that they were still active in their 90s and even after passing the century mark. Typical of these is Charles Bittner of Denver who was almost 101 as this was written. Each Sunday night, Charles spends the evening at Lakewood's Aviation Country Club dancing and enjoying dinner. Charles still stands tall and erect and prefers to spend his days working. Recently, he and his wife took a cruise to Alaska and they travel each winter to Arizona. Indicative of the many Lifex Constants that are part of his lifestyle and personality, Charles Bittner rarely worries, he does everything in moderation, he is invariably optimistic, and he never thinks about his age.

"He's great. He's so vivacious—and he's so quick," his wife Evelyn says. "He never stops to figure out an answer because he always has one. He's a joy to live with."

For most of us, it is merely our misconceptions that prevent us from emulating the Charles Bittners. We fail to appreciate that through cultivating health-building habits, we are extending our productive middle years, not our years of old age and senility.

The widely held concept that a long life must inevitably lead to sickness and senility destroys all incentive to extend our lives by upgrading our health. Hence it is not surprising to find that 40 percent of adult Americans continue to smoke, that one in two has some form of cardiovascular disease, that one male in five has a heart attack before reaching age 60, that one adult in three is overweight, and that one adult in twenty practices sound nutrition. Since it often takes a decade or more for the consequences of these habits to appear, lack of immediate feedback encourages individuals to continue undermining their health.

For millions of Americans, the stereotyped image that old age is synonymous with poor health remains a serious impediment to adopting any program for improved health or life extension.

Psychological Barriers to Life Extension

Another barrier is concern for what our friends and relatives might think if, instead of continuing to indulge, we suddenly began to take care of ourselves. These barriers are not insurmountable, as is demonstrated by hundreds of case histories of long-lived people who choose to adopt healthy lifestyles.

In fact, it is never too late to make the change. After suffering a severe heart attack at 87 and being told he would never walk again, Walter Casey Jones of Tacoma, Washington, went on a special diet and exercise program that dropped his weight by thirty-two pounds. He made a rapid recovery that he attributed to the many good health habits in his new lifestyle. Among them, he recommends such Lifex Constants as: never worry, develop a powerful will to live and never give up, be eternally optimistic, have fun, and eat a diet low in fat. These positive habits so transformed Jones's life that at age 102, he set out to tour the United States, driving his own motor home while he lectured to senior citizen groups about the benefits of the Lifex Constants. At age 109, the energetic Jones was still driving his own motor home and lecturing nationwide.

Can Nutritional Supplements Save Us from Bad Habits?

Some books suggest that by taking nutritional supplements we can remain healthy and long-lived while continuing to smoke, to eat a high-fat diet, to live in the fast lane, and to avoid all exercise. These unrealistic claims were arrived at by taking the results of animal lab studies published in scientific journals and extrapolating them into the context of human lives far beyond any reasonable expectation or observed result. Vitamins C and E possess certain anti-oxidant properties but they will not prevent lung cancer or heart disease. Nor does taking supplements to improve communication in the brain's neural pathways make us more intelligent. It simply improves conductivity in our neural pathways.

As Roy L. Walford, Ph.D., a pathologist at UCLA Medical School, stated in an interview in *U.S. News* on July 4, 1983, "Gerontology is filled with charlatans, quacks and even very good scientists gone awry."

So much misleading information has been published on longevity that people who are ready to make changes are confused about what to do to maximize their health. Much questionable "advice" is published by those who stand to profit from sale of foods, supplements, treatments, books or equipment, the benefits of most of which remain unproven.

This book promises no miracle foods, supplements or magic elixirs. The Lifex Constants which comprise the life extension program are based on an analysis of the lifestyles of more than a hundred thousand healthy, long-lived people.

Certainly, many healthy centenarians have one or two destructive habits. Some smoke (often without inhaling), others imbibe a few alcoholic drinks daily and some indulge in beverages containing caffeine. Seldom, however, do such harmful habits constitute more than 10 percent of all their lifestyle factors. When we examine the remaining 90 percent of their lifestyle profiles we invariably find they are filled with life-sustaining Constants.

The Common Denominators of Long Life

Lifex Constants are health-promoting habits and character traits that are repeated in the attitude and behaviors of healthful, long-lived people. These common denominators of good health complement each other and work to create a positive, health-oriented personality and lifestyle.

By analyzing evidence from a wide variety of lifestyle and population studies, researchers have now identified virtually all of the Lifex Constants and in many cases have produced a mathematical model of their statistical probability for extending life.

By making an overview of the findings of these studies, gerontologists have been able to assemble a composite of the many essentials for longevity. Thus, we now have a model showing how one may increase his or her chance of reaching a ripe old age in optimal health.

All the Lifex Constants were identified through objective studies which carefully excluded unproved theories, anecdotal sources or self-reporting by long-lived people themselves, and focused only on traits and habits that could be observed and verified. A brief review of some of these studies follows.

An Overview of Life Extension Studies

Among earlier, but still recent, studies was that of the Committee for an Extended Lifespan. After examining the profiles of over one thousand American centenarians, the Committee found that almost all shared five common traits: they did nothing to excess; most retired early and rose early; a huge proportion had strong spiritual faith; a large number were self-employed and enjoyed a high degree of personal autonomy; and most stayed busy all their lives.

Subsequent studies confirmed these same lifestyle constants and revealed others. In a study of one thousand long-lived people, Robert Samp, a physician at the University of Wisconsin, found that they shared such similarities as: possessing the flexibility to flow along with life's challenges instead of fighting them; avoiding prolonged stress; eating and drinking enjoyably but sparingly; retaining a keen interest in life and outside events; and keeping busy at either paid work or voluntary activities.

When Michael L. Cohen and Charles L. Rose examined the lives of five hundred males who died in 1965, they uncovered additional factors such as having few illnesses and a youthful appearance at 40 and over; never worrying; avoiding smoking; living in a rural environment; having a sense of humor; having a high occupational status; exercising regularly; and taking part in many social and recreational activities.

In 1969, Erdman B. Palmore, then professor of medical sociology at Duke University Medical Center, contributed several longevity factors from his thirteen-year longitudinal study. They include having a satisfying and useful work role; a high educational level; a higher income; great satisfaction with life; sound nutrition; and the ability to cope successfully with stress.

Many of these life extension factors were again confirmed in 1973 when the Social Security Administration released the results of its interviews with 1,130 American centenarians and added the axiom that we should develop a strong will to live.

A landmark in correlating the effects of lifestyle habits to longevity also occurred in 1973 when the Human Population Laboratory of the California

State Department of Health released the results of its eight-year study of seven thousand people in Alameda County. This important study, sponsored by the National Center for Health Research Services and Development, proved statistically that a 45-year-old male who practiced seven simple health-building habits could extend his life expectancy by eleven and one-half years.

From the study results, the researchers recommended these seven positive steps: avoid cigarette smoking; avoid excessive alcohol consumption; eat breakfast every day; maintain regular and moderate eating habits; keep your weight in proportion to your height; sleep at least seven but not more than eight hours each night; and take moderate exercise.

At age 45, males who practiced six or seven of the recommended steps were found to have a life expectancy of 33.08 more years compared to only 21.63 more years for those practicing fewer than four of the steps. By practicing all seven of these good health habits, a male aged 55 could increase his life expectancy by 11.25 years, at aged 65 by 7 years, and at age 75 by 4 years. Curiously, a 45-year-old woman following the seven steps increased her life expectancy by only 7 years. But at all ages, mortality among males observing the seven steps was barely one-sixth that of those who followed fewer than four steps.

Year by year, these studies gradually identified and verified the various Lifex Constants, and their results were being confirmed by similar studies in Japan, the Netherlands and elsewhere. In 1983, Dr. James Fries and his colleagues at Stanford University assembled a series of life-extending practices into a program designed to help people remain youthful and to experience quality living into their mid-80s. The steps recommended were: maintain strong ties with friends and family and cultivate social activity with people of all ages; join clubs and groups through which you can daily experience a variety of activities; stay mentally active and use your memory frequently; make bold, clear-cut choices and decisions; take complete charge of your life and remain independent; refrain from smoking or abusing alcohol or drugs; and take an abundance of physical exercise.

Supporting data for many Lifex Constants have also come from the National Institute of Aging's Baltimore Longitudinal Study (an ongoing twenty-five-year socio-behavioral investigation into the lives of eight hundred men and women) and the Framingham Heart Study which, since 1949, has identified most of the risks underlying heart disease.

More Pathways to Longer Life
Through making a composite of health-enriching factors among longevous communities such as the Seventh Day Adventists and the Mormons, other gerontologists have confirmed the effect of still other Lifex Constants.

[Although some interesting conclusions have also been drawn from studies in such reputed citadels of longevity as Vilcabamba (Ecuador), Hunza (Pakistan), South Africa, and the Russian Caucasus, almost all Lifex Constants were derived from studies of American centenarians who share cultural and geographic boundaries. (However, included are some studies made in nations where births and deaths have been reliably recorded for well over a century.)]

Three separate studies have probed into every aspect of the lifestyle of members of the SDA Church. A California study of 35,460 church members by Loma Linda University School of Medicine found that while only 2 percent were strict vegetarians, 20 percent did not eat most animal-derived foods and half the remainder were lacto-ovo vegetarians who abstained from all animal-derived foods but eggs and dairy products. The remainder tended to eat less meat and junk food than other Americans. Adventists also abstain almost completely from alcohol, tobacco and caffeine. Their philosophy also leads them away from many stressful activities commonly experienced by other Americans. Compared to the general California population, 70 percent fewer Adventists die of cancer, 68 percent fewer of respiratory diseases, 85 percent fewer of emphysema, 46 percent fewer of stroke, 60 percent fewer of heart disease, 93 percent fewer of cirrhosis of the liver, and 35 percent fewer from accidents. Similar studies of Adventists in the Netherlands and Denmark duplicated these findings and also confirmed significantly lower death rates from diabetes, bronchitis, peptic ulcer and uterine cancer.

In California, the life expectancy for a male Adventist between 35 and 40 is seven years longer than the average Californian. Those seven years are likely to be free of most dysfunctions associated with old age in the general population. When statistics were broken down to include only the authentically vegetarian Adventists, their life expectancy was found to be as much as eleven years or more in excess of the age-adjusted California average.

A study of church records of 15,500 California Mormons and 55,000 Utah Mormons was made in the late 1970s by James F. Enstrom of the UCLA Department of Public Health to identify cancer incidence. He compared the devout male Mormons who were active in their churches with the average male in the United States and found that the Mormons have a life expectancy seven years longer.

Further investigations showed that many strict Mormons have a life expectancy eleven or more years in excess of the national average. This has been ascribed to their adherence to the Mormon Words of Wisdom, a traditional health profile that forbids use of stimulants and drugs and recommends a diet largely based on vegetarian foods. Mormons who follow it are generally more highly educated than the average American; they consume barely one-third as much animal protein, and they tend to eat breakfast every day. Most Mormons still live uncomplicated lives in small towns and they seldom move. Mormons also rarely indulge in pre-marital or extra-marital intercourse and rarely divorce. They have large, stable families with many children and with a strong, multi-generation support system. The church also supplies financial security so that few Mormons ever need welfare. As a result, the death rate from smoking-related diseases in Utah is 60 percent below the average in the United States and the mortality rates for cancer, heart disease and cirrhosis of the liver are also much lower.

Similar results were found in a study of the Old Order Amish, who, although they eat a diet high in fat, live low-stress lives in stable and spiritual communities where they peform hard physical work. Here again, researchers found strict monogamy coupled with large and supportive multi-generation families. Although electricity, telephones and power-driven vehicles are absent, modern medical care is available and life is comfortable. As might be expected, the Amish life expectancy is also above average and incidence of cancer, cardiovascular and respiratory disease is low.

One Lifex Constant common to all three communities, of course, is strong spiritual faith. Yet the quality of life and health of these long-lived groups demonstrated that those willing to replace counterproductive habits with just a few Lifex Constants can readily extend their years of healthful activity.

We don't have to become athletic, religious, or make radical changes to achieve long life. Many centenarians merely take long, brisk daily walks for exercise. Many do not attend church but simply have faith in nature, love and people.

These conclusions might cause us to re-examine the benefits of what many Americans still regard as the "good life." Millions still spend their evenings and weekends chain smoking, consuming endless alcoholic beverages, and eating high-risk foods while avoiding all exercise and watching TV programs that often arouse stressful negative emotions.

For most of us, the elements involved in the "good life" are equally hazardous to health and longevity. Marbled steaks, coffee, cigarettes, ice cream, mechanization, luxury cars and soft living all add up to a disastrous threat to our health and life.

Through the program in this book, we can eliminate these risks and replace them with more enjoyable and more rewarding activities that have been scientifically shown to extend our lives and prolong our youth.

Road Map to Long Life

The purpose of this book is to put together all the discoveries and breakthroughs of life extension science into a single comprehensive program that anyone can use. It adapts the Lifex Constants so that we can create for ourselves the same basic personality and lifestyle found in the profiles of healthy, long-lived people. The Type-B Personality and the Wellness Lifestyle are explored in depth in Chapter 5.

The program is a systematic plan to enhance your wellness. It skips all ideas that are expensive, or that call for special treatments, equipment, drugs or exotic foods. It is based on simple methods designed to produce a healthier, happier and longer life.

First, you must obtain a complete understanding of the aging process. Only through knowing how the aging process actually works, and becoming familiar with the Lifex Constants, can we motivate ourselves toward transforming our health and acquiring the necessary skills and insight to do so.

How to Get Started

The first step is to carefully read this book through from beginning to end with special emphasis on Chapters 2, 3, 4, 5 and 6. As you read, you will find that the program unfolds chapter by chapter.

The second step is to put as many Lifex Constants to work as soon as possible.

After reading the entire book through for information, return to Chapter 5, which starts right off into the life extension program.

2

A Composite Theory of Aging

To learn how to live long, we must begin by understanding why most of us die prematurely. As an increasing flow of new information on biochemical and neurophysical aging mechanisms was released in recent years, a proliferation of aging theories appeared to explain how we age and why we die. Because the most dramatic discoveries concerned the interaction of particles, molecules and cells, theories based on the biochemical approach to aging prevailed.

Most biochemical theories begin with the formation of free radical damage resulting from intake of dietary fat and they explain aging in terms of DNA-error or cross-linkage. Other biochemical theories revolve around the hypothesized existence of a biological clock that programs obsolescence; or the accumulation of lipofuscin and other cellular waste.

These theories, which focus only on the genetic and cellular levels, have been criticized by prominent gerontologists on the grounds that aging cannot be satisfactorily explained within such narrow boundaries. Instead, researchers are finding that while these theories are still valid, they are simply minor functions in three more holistic theories that focus on the brain as the center of aging. These three widely accepted neurophysical theories are the Cholesterol, Stress and Immunological Theories of Aging.

Many gerontologists are also finding that both biochemical and neurophysical theories interact and interrelate so, in effect, they form a single unified theory that explains the entire aging process from free radicals to cells, organs, brains and personalities. As this chapter unfolds, it will become apparent that each theory blends with all others to form a single Composite Theory of Aging.

Biochemical Aging Theories

THE FREE RADICAL THEORY

Originated by Dr. Denham Harman of the University of Nebraska Medical School during the 1950s, the Free Radical Theory seeks to explain aging in terms of cellular damage that results from eating polyunsaturated fats in the diet. Free radicals are produced in living cells during oxidation of dietary fats when an electron is drawn away, leaving an atom or molecule that is unstable, chemically reactive, and capable of causing a wide range of damage to the cell's DNA, membrane and enzymes.

Free radicals can destroy the body's ability to synthesize prostacyclin, a prostaglandin [a hormone-like substance] essential for preventing blood clots. They can cause a decline in neurotransmitters, which link the brain's neural pathways and can lead to deterioration of the sensory nerves used in hearing, vision, smell and taste.

THE ERROR THEORY

The Error Theory explains aging in terms of the gradual accumulation and multiplying of errors in a cell's DNA (Deoxy-ribo-nucleic acid). DNA acts as a biochemical blueprint that comprises some three billion codings or letters that form our genes. Whenever a cell divides, a duplicate of this genetic blueprint is transferred to the offspring cell. Damage by free radicals, radiation, carcinogens, viruses or other toxins can cause slight errors in the codings so that instead of being a faithful copy of the original, the offspring is a mutation. As errors gradually accumulate and multiply, cells can become abnormal and cancerous or they can malfunction and cause gray hair, wrinkles, aging spots and a decline in the immune system.

Bernard L. Strehler of the University of Southern California, Los Angeles, has suggested that through the multiplication of errors as our cells divide, after age 30 most body functions begin to degenerate by 1 percent of their original capacity each year. This would bring our capacity to maintain life to an end at around age 117, which correlates exactly with the observed maximum limit of human life.

THE CROSS-LINKAGE THEORY

The Cross-Linkage Theory, originated by Dr. Johan Bjorksten and closely associated with the two preceding theories, explains aging as caused by oxidation processes that build harmful chemical bonds. This is also known as the Chemical Bridges Theory because the bonds bridge nucleic acids with large protein molecules and in the process destroy flexibility in the arteries, eye lens and skin. All over the body, collagen, a major component of human tissue, becomes rigid, destroying elasticity in skin and causing cartilage in joints to become brittle and hard. The most damaging effect is when Cross-Linkage affects the immune system's white cells so that they cease to defend the body.

OUR BUILT-IN BIOLOGICAL CLOCK

Biological clock theories explain aging in terms of a series of events such as puberty, menstruation, menopause, and male-pattern baldness that are programmed by a biological timing mechanism.

The Denckla Theory, originated by Dr. W. Donner Denckla of Harvard University Medical School in the late 1970s, postulates that aging changes are programmed through decreasing production by the pituitary gland of a substance called DECO. Through other glands and hormones, Dr. Denckla believes that DECO controls the basal metabolism of the entire body.

TOXEMIA

One prominent biochemical theory is that as we age, we fail to eliminate all of the body's waste products and they begin to cumulatively build up a condition of toxemia or self-poisoning. Through free radical and other activity, we accumulate brown pigment deposits of lipofuscin that appear as aging spots on the skin but are equally numerous throughout the body in neurons, muscles, organs and tissue.

Lipofuscin is caused by oxidation of polyunsaturated fats in the diet and by lack of exercise. In sedentary people who eat a high-fat diet, lipofuscin deposits can accumulate in neuron cells in the brain and elsewhere in the body.

Neurophysical Aging Theories

THE CHOLESTEROL THEORY OF AGING

Most researchers now agree that cholesterol blockages in the circulatory system, particularly in the arteries and capillaries, are the direct or indirect cause of most cardiovascular disease, which includes hypertension, heart disease and stroke. More than half of all Americans—over one million annually—die from one of these diseases, or from associated complications such as kidney disease and adult-onset diabetes.

Important discoveries in recent years have greatly extended our understanding of cardiovascular disease. Most of us are already aware that cholesterol, a saturated fat found in foods of animal origin, is one of the villains. Cholesterol, an alcohol classed as a sterol, is necessary for many body functions. It provides the nerves with their protective myelin sheath and every cell in the body requires cholesterol to absorb nutrients. Cholesterol, which looks like wax, has a melting point of 300 °F, making it solid at room temperature and insoluble at the body's temperature of 98.6 °F.

All indications are that early Homo sapiens and their ancestors were vegetarians. Since cholesterol exists only in foods of animal origin, our early primate ancestors had little, if any, cholesterol intake. But the greater the amount of vegetarian food our ancestors ate, the more cholesterol their cells required to absorb the nutrients. Thus, through evolution, the liver began to produce cholesterol in direct proportion to the amount of food we eat.

Today, our livers continue to synthesize cholesterol in proportion to the calories in the food we consume. However, because fat contains 9 calories per gram compared to only 4 calories for protein and between 2.75 and 4 for carbohydrates, a diet high in fat stimulates the liver to increase its cholesterol output by 30 percent or more. When the diet is high in foods of animal origin such as eggs, whole milk dairy products, red meat or fried foods, dietary cholesterol is added to the liver's cholesterol output, creating a huge cholesterol surplus.

Heavy meat eaters, for example, frequently consume 1,000 mgs of dietary cholesterol per day while the liver synthesizes another 3,000 mgs in response to the high calorie intake, making a total of 4,000 mgs. By comparison, the liver of a strict vegetarian who has no intake of cholesterol, may manufacture as little as 200 mgs of cholesterol per day. On average, the liver produces three or four times as much cholesterol as we consume in the diet.

The Subtle Pathology of Cholesterol Deposits

These destructive effects of cholesterol on our health and life expectancy have led some researchers to attribute most of the symptoms of aging to a pathology associated with the gradual accumulation of cholesterol deposits in our cardiovascular system. In people who consume saturated fats, atherosclerotic plaques frequently coat the entire arterial system. The larger the artery, the thicker the plaque. Studies show that artery walls thicken with age in direct proportion to increases in blood lipid levels and blood pressure. The table below illustrates how these increase with age in the average American.

Age	Average cholesterol level (mgs per dl)	Average blood pressure (mm Hg)
20	180–230	122/76
30	200–240	125/76
40	220–270	129/81
50	230–310	134/83
60	230–330	140/83
70	225–325	148/81

As cholesterol plaque thickens on artery walls, calcium ions react with fatty acids in the plaque to create a hard and almost indestructible coating on artery walls. Over the years, this process leads to arteriosclerosis or hardening of the arteries.

Gradually but imperceptibly, the insidious effects of cholesterol deposits choke off supplies of oxygen and nutrients to skin and hair cells, causing loss of elasticity and pliability. The skin begins to wrinkle and the hair begins to thin and turn gray. We lose suppleness in our joints and our reaction time slows. The capacity of our lungs and kidneys decline and our ability to perform physical work decreases. Altogether, scientists have attributed many of the common aging symptoms to the gradual accumulation of cholesterol.

New Light on Lipoproteins

Whether it originates in our diet or our liver, cholesterol is insoluble in the watery medium of the blood stream. To reach our cells, it must be transported by phospholipids, particles consisting of protein and lipid. The lipid content consists mostly of lecithin, which actually picks up and holds the cholesterol. The final combination of protein, lipid and cholesterol is known as lipoprotein.

Depending on the amount of lecithin it contains, a lipoprotein can be an LDL (low density lipoprotein) or an HDL (high density lipoprotein). The lower the density, the more lecithin the lipoprotein contains and the more cholesterol it can hold. LDL therefore carries three times as many cholesterol molecules as HDL. This makes LDL so unstable that it may drop some cholesterol during its passage through an artery or tiny capillary.

Free cholesterol so dropped possesses an affinity for endothelial cells, the skin cells of the smooth muscles that enclose our arteries. Smoking, emotional stress and a high level of blood cholesterol all create injuries to the lining of our arteries. Through these small injuries or tears in an artery wall, free cholesterol may attach itself to an endothelial cell. Once established, it attracts more free cholesterol. Eventually, an arterial plaque forms. As the plaque continues to grow, it increasingly occludes the flow of blood through the artery.

Plaques so formed are evenly distributed throughout the sixty thousand miles of arteries and capillaries that network the body. Eventually, plaques may occlude the coronary arteries causing angina pain or a heart attack; they may block a carotid artery causing a stroke; or they may restrict an artery in the leg causing severe claudication pain. Seldom are arterial plaques confined to a single artery. Thousands of persons who have had their occluded coronary arteries relieved through a by-pass operation have experienced a severe stroke a year or two later.

A variety of studies, including the Framingham Heart Study, have demonstrated that arterial plaques occur only in persons with such high-risk habits as eating a diet high in fat and protein; failing to exercise; smoking; and responding to stress in a destructive way. In people with these harmful habits, the liver synthesizes VLDLs (very low density lipoproteins), which pick up triglycerides and other fatty compounds derived from the fats and sugar we eat and transport them to various fat depositories in the body where they often serve to make us obese and overweight. The VLDLs are then transformed into the LDLs that initiate atherosclerosis (coating of the arteries by cholesterol deposits).

Based on animal studies made in 1981, Dr. Robert W. Mahley, a pathologist at the University of California, San Francisco, found that VLDL is produced only in response to a diet high in fat and cholesterol. Other researchers have shown that VLDL is also produced in response to an excessive calorie intake, which can only be achieved by overeating. There are now strong and growing indications that humans who eat sparingly of a diet low in fat and protein have a very low proportion of VLDLs and LDLs in their bloodstream, indicating that they are at low risk for heart disease.

Instead, such people have a high proportion of HDLs. HDLs carry only one-third as much cholesterol as LDLs, making them extremely stable. In fact, HDLs actively seek more cholesterol to carry. HDLs accomplish this by carrying the enzyme LCAT (lecithin-cholesterol-acyl-transferase) which, in the presence of Vitamin C, dissolves cholesterol deposits in artery walls. The free cholesterol combines with lecithin in the HDLs and is transported to the kidneys, where it is excreted as bile.

Put more simply, HDLs block the uptake of cholesterol into artery walls and gradually remove the plaques; consequently, the higher our HDL level, the lower our risk of atherosclerosis and other cardiovascular disease.

Is Dietary Fat Really Dangerous?

This discovery, made only a few years ago, solved a controversy among cardiologists. As far back as the 1950s, researchers had correlated high levels of cholesterol in the bloodstream (serum cholesterol) with an increasing risk of heart disease. The Framingham Study revealed that a cholesterol level of 250 (mgs per deciliter) carried three times the risk of heart disease as did a level below 194. Since the norm for Americans in their 40s is 245, this meant that the majority of Americans, especially males, were at risk for cardiovascular disease.

For years thereafter, Americans were exhorted by press, radio and books to reduce their intake of saturated (animal) fat, to cut out smoking, and to exercise more. This advice, which emanated from such influential sources as the United States government, the Framingham Study and the American Heart Association, led to a decline in heart disease of 25 percent during the ten-year period between 1968 and 1979. In England, by contrast, where both the medical profession and the public remained apathetic to lifestyle changes, the cardiovascular mortality rate remained unchanged.

Many Americans, however, resented these dietary changes and challenged researchers by pointing out that a significant proportion of people who ate a high-fat diet had a low serum-cholesterol level. Others had a high serum-cholesterol level but experienced no sign of cardiovascular disease. It was also discovered that several important studies had failed to find a relationship between high cholesterol levels and heart disease.

Articles soon began to appear reassuring us that we had been misled and that, after all, it was perfectly safe to go on eating high-fat foods, especially eggs, which have a high lecithin content.

Low-Risk Populations

Meanwhile, population studies continued to show that in vegetarian societies, and in countries where little fat or animal protein is eaten, the incidence of cardiovascular disease remained low. A 1979 study by the South African Institute for Medicine revealed, for example, that atherosclerosis, heart disease and stroke were rare among men and women of the Tswanas, a tribe living within one hundred miles of Johannesburg where whites have a high level of heart disease. Blood analysis showed that the HDL level of Tswana people was exceptionally high and that it remained high throughout life. The total absence of cardiovascular disease was confirmed by Dr. Gabriel Roux, superintendent of the George Stegman Mission Hospital that serves 250,000 people in the area.

Researchers who conducted the study attributed the Tswanas's complete freedom from heart disease to their relaxed lifestyle and freedom from stress, their lifelong devotion to physical activity and their diet of cereals, legumes, fruit and vegetables. Only 13 percent of their calories are derived from fat and only one-third of that is from animal sources. The average American derives 38 percent of all calories from fat of which some two-thirds is from animal sources.

New Barometer of Heart Disease Risk

The controversy was finally ended when investigators for the Framingham Heart Study discovered that the ratio between total cholesterol and HDLs gave a far more dependable assessment of heart disease risk than that based on using the cholesterol level alone. By dividing the total cholesterol level by the HDL level, the following risk ratio averages were obtained for differentiated groups.

Control group	Risk ratio
Newborn baby	2.3
Strict vegetarian	2.8
One-half average risk	3.4
Marathon runners	3.4
Active female bicyclists	3.6
Moderately active bicyclists	3.9
Average female risk (United States)	4.4
Average male risk (United States)	5.00
Average male heart disease victim	5.4
Twice average female risk (United States)	7.1
Twice average male risk (United States)	9.6

Through this important discovery, anyone can now assess his or her risk of heart disease or stroke from physical causes. Although it may be available only through your doctor, many medical labs now offer this lipid analysis called Heart Disease Risk Profile.

Through the Cholesterol:HDL Ratio we now know why some people with a high total-cholesterol are relatively safe from heart attack. The reason is that they also have a high HDL level. For example, a person with a high total-cholesterol level of 255 mgs per deciliter—previously considered to be at risk for heart disease—but with an equally high HDL level of 75, has a ratio of only 3.4 which is exactly half the average person's risk for heart disease.

Conversely, a person with a total cholesterol level of only 160 and an HDL level of 30 has a ratio of 5.3 and may be at risk of heart disease.

LDL levels, also available through the same blood analysis profile, provide further evidence of heart disease risk. A level of 125 mgs per deciliter is considered normal for a 45-year-old male; 115 mgs is considered normal for a 45-year-old female. Higher readings indicate increased risk.

Hence, the lower our cholesterol level and the higher our HDL level, the lower our risk of heart disease. We can improve our Cholesterol:HDL Ratio in two ways. First, by eating a diet low in fat and animal protein and high in natural vegetarian foods and Vitamin C. Second, by exercising regularly, which raises our HDL level.

As a case in point, Andrew Ferguson, a Denver businessman, found he had a cholesterol level of 240 and an HDL level of only 48, making a ratio of 5. Cardiologists consider anyone with a ratio of 4.5 or higher to be at risk of heart disease. Andrew immediately reduced his fat intake from 40 percent of his daily calorie intake to only 5 percent. He began to swim for half a mile five times a week. In three months, his ratio had been reduced to a safe 3.5.

Angina, Heart Attack and Stroke

Both angina and heart attack are caused when a cholesterol plaque blocks a coronary artery that supplies oxygen-bearing blood to the heart muscle. When the heart is deprived of oxygen for a short period, the condition is known as angina pectoris, a sensation of tightness, pressure, choking and squeezing in the chest, left arm and sometimes the lower jaw. The symptoms usually disappear when the victim rests. Injury to the heart is slight and the damage is reversible.

If blood flow to the heart is reduced for longer than a few minutes, the heart muscle begins to turn blue for lack of oxygen and begins to die. When only a small area dies, the victim usually recovers and the area becomes scar tissue. If a large area of heart muscle dies, or a vital area of the heart is affected, a myocardial infarction, or heart attack, occurs and the victim may die.

Neither angina nor heart attack are actually diseases of the heart but are caused by a restricted flow of blood through the coronary arteries. In most cases, the heart itself is perfectly sound.

A stroke occurs when the flow of oxygen-bearing blood to the brain is cut off or reduced. Sixty-five percent of strokes are classified as *thrombotic* and are caused when a blood clot becomes jammed in a main artery already partially blocked by atherosclerosis. Most other strokes result from a hemorrhage due to a ruptured artery or to an aneurism (a balloon-like weakness in the artery wall). Both types are caused by a cholesterol build-up in the artery and are often triggered by hypertension (high blood pressure) or by stress.

Some people have a series of very small strokes caused by a cholesterol blockage, a blood clot in an arteriole (a tiny artery) or by a temporary blockage in a larger artery. Damage from these is usually not serious, however, a more severe stroke can destroy functioning brain tissue with resulting loss of muscle-movement control, usually on one side of the body only, and a loss of ability to speak.

Hypertension is another symptom of heart disease that often results from atherosclerosis. As cholesterol plaques build up in the arteries, the space available for blood is reduced. As a result, the blood is squeezed under pressure into a smaller area.

In another part of the cardiovascular system, cholesterol plaque waterproofs lymph vessel walls, inhibiting transport of waste products from cells. Toxic wastes build up in the cells, creating a condition of toxemia that gradually poisons the tissues. Toxic cells then release enzymes called cathepsins, which begin to slowly destroy the body's tissues and organs by autolysis.

THE STRESS THEORY OF AGING

Cardiovascular diseases like angina, heart disease, stroke and hypertension are also frequently triggered by stress. Hypertension, for instance, results when the smooth muscles, which surround each artery and capillary, constrict and compress the blood into a smaller volume, thereby raising its pressure. Most hypertension is due to a combination of atherosclerosis and artery constriction and, in many cases, an excessive consumption of salt. (Salt increases the body's water content, creating greater pressure on arterial blood vessels.)

Artery constriction is part of the Fight or Flight response, a mechanism triggered by the hypothalamus gland whenever we perceive a situation as threatening. With hair-trigger speed, it readies the body to meet immediate physical danger. The sympathetic nervous system, the emergency branch of the autonomic nervous system, takes over and all systems are GO. Epeniphrine and cortisol squirt into the bloodstream to speed up body functions, including the heart rate, and to increase circulation. Stomach acid production increases as blood is shunted from the digestive system to muscles and brain.

In preparation for a possible wound, the clotting ability of the blood increases and red blood cells pour into the bloodstream to carry additional oxygen to the muscles. Meanwhile, white blood cell production is cut back, suppressing the immune system. Glycogen (sugar) is released from the liver, causing the blood sugar level to soar and our muscles fill with energy, and tense for action. Finally, the autonomic nerve fibers, which parallel each blood vessel, signal receptors in the smooth muscles to constrict every artery and capillary.

The result? Blood pressure shoots up immediately. This instinctive response to a threat to our survival prepared us during the Stone Age to combat or to flee from a physical threat. But the hypothalamus gland cannot distinguish whether a perceived threat is physical or psychological. It turns on the same Fight or Flight response whether the threat is actual or imagined. In either case, it leaves us with our muscles all tensed up for instant action and with our mind prepared to face a hostile world.

In primitive society, we might have dispelled this tension and attitude by either fighting for our life or by using our tensed-up energy to run away, and our blood pressure would swiftly drop back to normal. However, in modern society, we can frequently do neither. So we remain filled with tension and we continue to feel that the world is a threatening, unfriendly place. Our blood pressure remains elevated for as long as these conditions last.

In today's stressful world, many of us live in an unbroken state of emergency with a low-level Fight or Flight response smoldering continually. Our arteries become permanently constricted and we experience chronic hypertension. Since it reflects both our physical and psychological condition, blood pressure is an important predictor of death from heart disease, and is a dependable barometer of our life expectancy.

Blood Pressure—Key to Long Life

Blood pressure is measured by taking the systolic pressure, the heart's contracting phase, during which the blood in the chambers is forced onward; and the diastolic pressure, the resting phase during which the chambers are filling with blood. If the systolic pressure reads 120 (mm Hg) and the diastolic 80, the pressure is stated as "120 over 80" and is written 120/80, which is the normal pressure for a healthy adult.

Any reading under 140/90 is considered normal. Most healthy centenarians have had a systolic pressure of 120 or slightly below for most of their lives and a diastolic pressure of 70 or slightly less. By comparison, a diastolic pressure of 105 or above indicates four times the risk of heart disease as a reading of 75 or below. A systolic of 150 indicates twice the risk of heart attack as a reading of 120 and a systolic of 160 indicates four times the risk.

Insurance companies have translated readings into direct predictions of life expectancy. A pressure of 140/95 indicates a life expectancy nine years shorter than a person with a pressure of 120/80 or less. A reading of 150/100 indicates that normal life expectancy may be reduced by sixteen and one-half years.

Most physicians classify a person as hypertensive with a reading of 150/95. In the Framingham Study, hypertensive men aged over 45 developed three times more heart attacks and seven times more strokes than normotensive men.

You can easily measure your own blood pressure by purchasing a blood pressure kit from a drugstore or medical supply outlet. Most reliable, and strongly recommended to anyone with normal hearing, is the mercury column type. A kit, along with a stethoscope, should cost about $65. This is less than the cost of three visits to the doctor's office for a blood-pressure check. In a single evening, you can learn to take your own blood pressure.

Taking your own blood pressure is a recommended step for anyone with a tendency to hypertension. Cardiologists have found that when a nurse or doctor takes a person's blood pressure, the excitement and nervousness of being in a clinical setting always elevates the blood pressure and frequently sets off a low-level Fight or Flight response, causing blood pressure to soar. This temporary deviation in blood pressure during examination is known as "labile hypertension." A temporary rise in blood pressure can also occur after any stressful event in a person's life. Yet the rest of the time, blood pressure may be normal.

Some heart specialists believe that 25 percent of all persons diagnosed as hypertensive are merely labile. Labile hypertension may also occur while having your blood pressure taken by a machine in a drugstore when other people are watching.

Among many surveys proving that home readings are more accurate is a 1979 study conducted at the University of Washington, Seattle. When sixty hypertensives learned to take their own blood pressure readings, 43 percent showed a drop of ten points on either systolic or diastolic or both, while 57 percent reported lesser reductions. A ten-point drop accomplishes what most hypertensive drugs can achieve.

One can only guess at how many hundreds of thousands of labile Americans have been incorrectly diagnosed as having high blood pressure. Many have been placed on anti-hypertensive drugs, a type of medication with many complex side effects. Through taking your own blood pressure, you can eliminate this risk.

Our Thoughts Influence Our Health

Increasing scientific evidence is revealing that every organ in the body is connected to the brain and that aging is paced by changes in brain chemistry. For instance, the brain governs most body functions, either through the pathways of the central nervous system or through the neuro-endocrine axis, which releases hormones that control our glands.

Researchers on organs such as the heart must refocus their studies to include the brain. Frequently, the seat of heart disease lies in the brain rather than in the heart.

The ultimate control over the body's physiology lies in the way we think. There is increasing evidence that our thoughts trigger feelings that directly influence the body's entire physiology, especially the cardiovascular, immune, nervous and digestive systems.

Each year, tens of thousands of people are stricken with cancer a few weeks or months after their minds have reacted negatively to a cluster of disturbing life events. Their negative thoughts trigger negative emotions that translate into suppressing the body's immune system, our defense against cancer and infectious disease. When oncologist O. Carl. Simonton taught 159 patients with terminal cancer to reverse their feelings by visualizing positive thoughts and images, 26 experienced significant regression or complete remission of their cancer while in 14 others the disease remained stable.

From these and hundreds of similar experiments and discoveries, gerontologists have concluded that personality is the key to a long and healthy life.

Stress Is Everywhere

Personality determines our response to stress. Stress is anything that makes it difficult to cope with life's changes. Some years ago, Doctors Thomas Holmes and Richard Rahe of the University of Washington Medical School measured the average person's response to the stress of such disturbing life events as death of a spouse, divorce, separation, illness or injury, loss of a job, or financial problems. It was found that whenever such crises occur in a cluster, they tend to overload our circuits and our emotional fuses blow. Based on the number of life crises that had occurred in the previous twelve months, Doctors Holmes and Rahe were able to predict, with a high degree of accuracy, the risk of subsequent physical illness.

Since then, other researchers have found that such everyday stresses as continual noise, congestion, confusion, freeway driving, absorbing new information, meeting deadlines, overwork, conflicts of all kinds, and job insecurity all create changing conditions to which we must constantly adjust.

Intermittent stress is less harmful because the mind calms down as soon as the source of stress ceases, and the body quickly recovers; however, a continual series of stresses, or a cluster, allows no let up during which the body's powers of resilience can rebound and recover. Hence, in today's fast-paced world, stress is more complex and pervasive and its effects become cumulative and chronic.

Long-Lived People Flow with Stress

Investigations show that healthy, long-lived people are able to adjust successfully to life's changes by being flexible and flowing along with the changes rather than resisting them. Through this positive attitude, they transform stress into non-stress. Most of us, by comparison, interpret change as threatening and hostile and we resist it.

In doing so, we invoke negative feelings such as worry, fear, anger, frustration, and anxiety. Each of these aggressive emotions may trigger the Fight or Flight response. This, in turn, releases CRF (cortocotropin releasing factor), which plays a dominant role in translating psychological stress into physiological changes. CRF promotes release of ACTH from the pituitary gland, which stimulates the adrenal glands to produce more hormones. Among them is cortisol, which directly suppresses the immune system. CRF may also stimulate release of catecholamines like adrenalin or noradrenalin, which can alter heart rate and blood pressure. Also released are hormones that affect the gastrointestinal tract leading to stress diseases such as ulcers or ulcerative colitis. Through these subtle chemical changes, stress can have a profound effect on our health and longevity.

Using new diagnostic equipment available only recently, scientists have discovered that heart attacks can be induced by mechanisms other than blocked coronary arteries. Artery spasm and platelet clumping are functions of the Fight or Flight state, which can occur within seconds of experiencing severe emotional stress. Both conditions are also severely aggravated by cigarette smoking. These newly discovered forms of heart disease often occur in combination with atherosclerosis; they may also occur independently.

How Stress Harms Us Directly

Stress causes a decline in production of the immune system's white cells, which reduces the body's resistance to infectious diseases and cancer. A 1977 study at Texas A&M University clearly demonstrated that most cancer patients have experienced almost twice as many emotional upsets in life as people who have not had cancer. Other studies confirm that most cancer patients have undergone massive emotional crises within the previous six to twenty-four months.

At any time, when emotional stress increases, it may overstimulate the sympathetic nervous system and intensify arterial muscle contraction, leading to a condition called artery spasm. Artery spasm can squeeze the coronary arteries so tightly that blood flow to the heart is restricted and angina pains occur. When coronary spasm occurs in arteries already partially blocked by cholesterol, the heart's pacemaker mechanism becomes electrically unstable, giving way to ventricular fibrillation, a wildly uncontrolled arrythmia in which the heart beats so chaotically that no blood is pumped. Sudden cardiac death—a form of heart attack—may then occur. However, in 27 percent of all cases of sudden cardiac death, the victim has no significant cholesterol blockage and the heart is sound.

This discovery is vitally important because researchers are finding that 60 percent of heart attack victims die not from myocardial infarction, resulting from cholesterol blockage alone, but from sudden cardiac death, a condition invariably triggered by the quality of our thoughts.

The associated form of angina, also triggered by harmful negative thinking, is known as Prinzmetal's Angina or Variant A. Angina. It occurs most commonly in men between ages 20 and 50 but is becoming increasingly common in women of all ages who smoke. Physicians dislike this unstable form of angina because they have no medicine to control our thoughts. Instead, they often prescribe a beta blocker to block the beta receptors through which the nervous system activates the artery muscles.

Studies by Dean Ormish, M.D., of Harvard Medical School, have shown that through calming the mind with meditation, attacks of this form of angina can be reduced by 90 percent or more with a corresponding reduction in risk of sudden cardiac death.

Depending on body chemistry, negative thoughts may also stimulate nerve endings in the intestines, leading to an ulcer or ulcerative colitis. Both are regarded as stress-caused diseases.

Stress may also lead to platelet clumping through increasing the blood's ability to clot. One function of the Fight or Flight response is to minimize bleeding at a wound site during possible combat. A pair of prostaglandins work in tandem to produce the coagulating quality of blood platelets. Prostacyclin dilates the arteries and prevents platelets clumping and sticking to artery walls while Thromboxane A_2 causes arteries to constrict and platelets to clump.

Thromboxane A_2 is produced by the platelets themselves, either in response to stress or in response to a high fat diet. In a person with healthy arteries, the platelets drift through the capillaries in single file, carrying oxygen and nutrients to tissue and muscle; however, in a person who eats a diet high in fats, and who may already have cholesterol blockage, additional fat in the bloodstream neutralizes the electrical charges that keep the platelets separated. In this way, fat acts like sludge, causing platelets to become sticky and to adhere to each other.

When additional Thromboxane A_2 is activated during a period of stress, the platelets actually clump together. Through clumping, their oxygen bearing capacity is reduced. The clumps become lodged at bends in the capillaries, cutting off oxygen and nutrients to body cells and creating fatigue.

Large clumps may aggregate inside a coronary artery, and in conjunction with a cholesterol plaque or artery spasm, they may narrow or completely close the artery. The result may be angina, myocardial infarction or sudden cardiac death. Clumping can also block an artery in the leg causing painful claudication, or an artery in the neck, causing a stroke.

Additional studies have shown that a secondary effect of Thromboxane A_2 is to cause constriction of artery walls. Production of Thromboxane A_2 is also boosted by the male hormone testosterone, which means that men are more prone to blood clotting and artery spasm than women.

Stress may damage artery walls through secretion of the steroid hormone cortisol during the Fight or Flight response. A study by Eugene Sprague, Ph.D., of the University of Texas, showed that when monkeys were given a large daily dose of cortisol together with a high cholesterol diet, they developed twice as much artery damage as a group of monkeys given a high cholesterol diet alone. This landmark study was the first to show a direct correlation between stress and artery damage. Additional artery damage may occur through artery spasm and smoking.

How Stress Harms Us Indirectly

When we react to a stressful change with an inappropriate response, we feel tense and uneasy. As a result, we often attempt to pacify our negative emotions by indulging in destructive habits. We seek relief by smoking cigarettes; drinking beverages containing caffeine; taking excessive amounts of alcohol; compulsively eating junk food or high-risk foods; taking drugs such as tranquilizers and sedatives; or by failing to exercise.

Yielding to such habits engenders a helpless, pessimistic attitude through which we lose control of our life and health. We eat, drink and smoke in response to stress.

The late Hans Selye, a pioneer in stress research, described aging as the cumulative result of all the stress encountered during a lifetime. Many specialists today are finding that the cumulative chronic stress of our high-tech lifestyle is the primary cause of most disease. For those unable to cultivate the flexibility to flow with stress, the rapid pace and unrelenting demands of today's business world can accelerate aging. Because our capacity to tolerate stress diminishes with age, this type of stress is particularly hard on us as we grow older.

According to the American Academy of Family Physicians, two-thirds of all office visits to family physicians are prompted by stress-related dysfunctions. Another survey by S. J. Breiner of Michigan State University concluded that at least 40 percent of all men and women die of diseases that are triggered in the mind. Thus, it is not surprising to learn that inability to cope with stress has been identified as a major cause of all types of cardiovascular disease, ulcers, cancer, kidney disease, diabetes, rheumatoid arthritis, leukemia, asthma, ulcerative colitis, allergies, backache, psoriasis, eczema, prolapsed stomach and intestines, sterility and chronic anxiety and depression. Long periods of poor nutrition and other negative habits lay the groundwork for each of these dysfunctions. But the immediate cause is unresolved stress.

THE IMMUNOLOGICAL THEORY OF AGING

Developed by Dr. Roy Walford and by other immunologists, this theory traces many of the dysfunctions of aging to the gradual deterioration and malfunctioning of the body's immune system.

The immune system consists of some 126 billion lymphocyte (white) cells. Approximately 70 percent of these are T-cells, named because they are produced in the thymus gland, an apple-sized gland located at the base of the neck. The remaining 30 percent are B-cells, produced in bone marrow.

T-cells patrol the bloodstream on a constant surveillance mission to detect invading bacteria, virus or any other non-self cells and, if found, to alarm the rest of the immune system. T-cells can recognize any other cell by the antigen (molecular recognition code) on its surface. When a T-cell encounters an invading foreign cell, or any other non-self cell, it memorizes the invader's antigen. The T-cell then speeds to the closest lymph gland where B-lymphocytes and killer T-cells gather.

Here, the messenger T-cell alerts killer lymphocytes that hasten to the site of the foreign invader. The messenger then begins touching each B-cell, causing the production of antibodies. Antibodies are protein molecules which bind to the antigen of a non-self cell, marking it for destruction by lymphocytes and scavenger cells called phagocytes. Within minutes, the non-self cell has been tagged by antibodies and becomes the target of attack by an army of white cells spewing complement and other enzymes that pierce fatal holes in the invader's cell wall.

Body cells, which through mutation become neoplasms (cancer cells) are recognized as non-self as are the bacteria and viruses of infectious diseases. (Viruses are recognized only after they occupy a body cell.) These non-self cells can then survive only when the lymphocytes fail to match their antigen. This can happen through immunological overload when the total number of invading bacteria plus neoplasms outnumber the immune system's capacity, or when the immune system's function is suppressed by stress or by aging. In either case, the immune system is unable to mount a counter attack, leaving cancer cells to multiply and form a tumor; or infections like influenza or pneumonia to multiply out of control.

Research in recent years has revealed that the immune system deteriorates as we grow older due to the gradual disappearance of the thymus gland. By age 35, the thymus has virtually disappeared in people who smoke, overeat, or who indulge in other high-risk habits. As the thymus gradually shrinks, so does production of thymosin, a hormone essential for normal functioning of T-cells. Without sufficient thymosin, T-cells lose their aggressiveness towards non-self cells. Instead, they may become abnormal and attack the body's own cells. This process, called auto-immunity, is responsible for a variety of auto-immune diseases such as rheumatoid arthritis and purpura.

Through animal experiments, Walford and others have demonstrated that in aging animals treated with thymosin, T-cells regained their health and vigor

3

How to Compensate for Genetic Handicaps to Life Extension

Sir William Oslev, a famous British physician, once stated that, "the way to live a long life is to contract a chronic disease and take good care of it." During his long career, Sir William had observed hundreds of patients who, after finding themselves stricken with a chronic disease, had become so frightened at the thought of dying that they had transformed their life-style habits and adopted many of the Lifex Constants. In spite of their diabetes, bronchitis or emphysema, they had still managed to outlive their life expectancy.

The same philosophy can be used to offset genetic factors such as sex, and blood type, which can affect our life expectancy. Although we cannot change these factors with which we were endowed at birth, by learning to compensate for them, we can still outlive our peers by many years.

The American Black's Crossover Phenomenon
The stress of being black in America makes blacks twice as susceptible as whites to hypertension and reduces life expectancy by five to eight years. (Blacks in Africa, by contrast, have an extremely low level of heart disease.)

From age 75 on, the life expectancy of American blacks begins to exceed that of whites and the greater the age, the greater the crossover differential in favor of blacks. Dr. Johan Bjorksten, a prominent gerontologist, has explained it in terms of skin pigmentation. Black or brown skin screens out most ultra-violet and other cosmic radiation, which is a primary cause of cell mutation and cross-linkage. As a result, the percentage of American black centenarians is well in excess of their demographic representation.

People Live Longer with Type O Blood

Professor Gerhard Joergensen of West Germany has found that, statistically, people with Type O blood have a 60 percent better chance of reaching age 75 than those with Type A blood. Forty-four percent of the population has Type O blood.

First-Born Children Are Longer-Lived

First-born children tend to achieve a higher socio-economic level in life and to outlive their siblings by up to one year. This phenomenon is believed to be partly due to the mother's younger age. The earlier in the birth order of siblings, the longer the life expectancy. However, children born to a mother in the 18 to 35 age bracket tend to outlive those born to a mother under 18 or over 35. First-born children are also high achievers, leading to higher educational and occupational levels, all of which are Lifex Constants.

Heredity

When identical twins Lucy Brown Coleman and Elizabeth Brown English, both of McRae, Georgia, reached age 101 in 1983, gerontologists estimated the odds of identical twins living to the century mark as one in 700 million. Since identical twins develop from the same fertilized egg and share the same genetic inheritance, this would seem to reduce the influence of heredity on long life.

Various studies have also failed to show any significant correlation between heredity and long life. A Gallup Poll of nonegarians in the United States found that 49 percent had no parent who lived beyond 80; 29 percent had neither a sibling nor parent who lived past 80; 19 percent had no blood relative at all who lived past 80. Another study by Dr. Robert Samp at the University of Wisconsin, funded by the American Council of Life Insurance, found that heredity and chromosome factors had little influence on longevity after 30. Still another study at Duke University's Center for the Study of Aging found that after we reach age 60, the ages to which our parents lived has little influence on our own life expectancy. The study found that after reaching 60, the best indicators for long life are satisfaction with work and volunteer activities and ability to function physically.

While heart disease, hypertension and adult-onset diabetes seem to run in families, most gerontologists believe this is due not to inherited genes but to children having learned from their parents the same self-destructive habits of eating, living and thinking which caused these diseases in the parents.

Likewise, the long-lived offspring of long-lived parents appear to owe their success more to having learned about the Lifex Constants from their parents than to inheriting any specific gene.

Some less common diseases may occasionally be inherited; however, in almost all cases, our personality and lifestyle have far greater influence on longevity than heredity.

Why Women Outlive Men

Throughout the world, in most societies and cultures, women outlive men by an average 7.8 years. Until 1983, it was assumed that this indicated a genetic and hormonal basis for superior female longevity. In 1983, however, a study of 8,300 men and women in Erie County, Pennsylvania, by Dr. Gus Miller of Pennsylvania's Indiana University, and Dean R. Gerstein of the National Research Council, revealed that women's longevity lead is primarily due to a higher incidence of smoking, accidents, homicide and suicide among males. In societies where these risks for men are absent, men live approximately as long as women. Doctors Miller and Gerstein confirmed this through a survey of 4,000 men and women in an Amish community where smoking, homicide, suicide and accidents were rare. Under these conditions, they found that men generally lived as long as women. Several studies of similar societies around the world confirm these results.

This exciting new information means that men who do not smoke or expose themselves to risk of violent death have a life expectancy equal to that of women in general. Confirming this trend is a gradual narrowing of the male-female longevity differential as women increasingly enter the stress of the business world. This diminishing differential is particularly noticeable among more highly educated couples where the male becomes aware of the benefits of exercising, quitting smoking, and eliminating fat and animal protein from the diet.

At present, however, the average American woman still faces seven years of widowhood and by age 65, for every 1,000 women only 650 men remain alive. Among women themselves, those who have born three children live longest while childless women, those who have born only one child, or those who have born seven or more children live fewest years. Women of today age more slowly than their mothers or grandmothers through enjoying greater personal freedom, fewer and safer pregnancies and childbirth, and the opportunity for self-actualization through work outside the home.

Prior research had ascribed the female lead in longevity to several biological causes. Women, for instance, have two X-chromosomes compared to an X and a Y chromosome in men, giving them a more vigorous and protective immune system (but also one that is more prone to auto-immune disease). Meanwhile, HDL levels remain high in women until age 50 while men experience a sharp 15 percent decline soon after reaching puberty.

This is attributed to production of the male hormone testosterone, which predisposes men toward heart disease. Several studies have found that men castrated early in life and, therefore, deprived of testosterone, outlive other men by 11 to 14 years and even outlive women by an average 6.7 years. Testosterone stimulates the liver to produce more LDL while estrogen, the female hormone, stimulates production of HDL. The testosterone effect also regulates the prostaglandin balance, placing men at risk of heart disease through blood clotting or artery spasm. This tendency is helped by women's smaller size, lower metabolic rate and generally lower blood pressure.

Men also traditionally lead more aggressive and competitive lives and many follow such traditions as smoking, heavy drinking, taking unnecessary risks, suppressing emotions, following dangerous occupations and eating a high-fat, high-protein diet. As a result, men still lead women in fourteen of the fifteen leading causes of death in the United States.

Compensating for Genetic Factors

We cannot do much about changing our heredity or sex, but we do not have to become a victim of genetics. These factors can be easily offset by adopting two or three Lifex Constants. Were all men to quit smoking and to avoid risk of violent death, for instance, the statistical female longevity lead would vanish. Again, merely by following the seven good health habits recommended by the California State Department of Health (see "An Overview of Life Extension Studies" in Chapter 1), a middle-aged male can increase his life expectancy by eleven and one-quarter years, more than compensating for any genetic factors.

To sum it all up: far from being handicap, a potentially life-shortening genetic handicap can easily become the focus through which you can extend your life far beyond your average life expectancy.

4

The Stages of Aging

From birth to death, men and women progress through five general stages of aging. How rapidly we travel through each stage depends on the extent to which we indulge in, or abstain from, health-destroying habits. After reaching age 20, those who believe in a short life may find that each stage is brief. For those who recognize that quality living can extend into their ninth decade or later, each stage may occupy twenty years or more.

The First Stage of Life: Birth to Age 20

Incredibly, life-shortening risks appear in the lives of American children soon after weaning. To appease their children, parents too often reward them with snacks and they learn to eat for entertainment rather than to relieve hunger. Then, from an early age, children who observe their parents leading sedentary lives will assume a similar lifestyle as they grow older.

A study of 42,444 children conducted in 1982 by the American Health Foundation found that 20 percent of the youngsters were obese; 25 percent regularly ate foods high in fats and cholesterol; 11 percent smoked cigarettes; 22 percent had drunk alcohol within the previous two weeks (their average age was twelve); and 31 percent reported that at home, their meals were salted despite widespread cautions in the media against the use of salt.

Many American teenagers get insufficient exercise to raise their HDL levels high enough to dissolve their cholesterol plaques. In one test, American teenagers failed 71 percent of physical fitness tests in comparison to a failure rate of only 20 percent by Russian youngsters.

Compared with records from a century ago, today's American teenagers are growing taller and heavier on diets loaded with meat, milk and sugar. Each American, on average, consumes 130 pounds of sugar per year compared with just 10 pounds a hundred years ago. A century ago, the average American woman reached puberty between 15 and 17. On today's high-fat, high-protein, high-sugar diet, one-third of American girls reach puberty before age 11.

In young people who eat more food than their bodies need, whose diet is high in fats, eggs, dairy foods, meat and refined carbohydrates (sugar and white flour), a progressive loss of body function and intellectual ability has already set in by their twentieth birthday.

Because the functional capacity of body organs in young adults is between four and ten times that required to maintain life, these effects go unnoticed. But from an early age, most of us begin to acquire a personality and lifestyle that erode our health.

The Second Stage of Life: Ages 20 to 40

All aging theories are based on the second law of thermodynamics which states, in essence, that any organization or structure will begin to undergo spontaneous destruction unless energy is spent on maintaining it. Soon after age 20, most of us begin to slowly disintegrate. As body protein is replaced by fat, inactive people begin to lose 3 to 5 percent of their muscles, glands and organs with each ensuing decade.

We are still tall and strong at 30 and most of us have 20/20 vision but signs of degeneration are evident. As we try to compete on the job and to cope with time pressures and deadlines, our responses to stressful life events translate into unnatural stresses on our bodies. Lines begin to appear on our foreheads. By age 30, most American adults have abandoned all strenuous exercise. One result is that the supply of blood to each liter of muscle tissue has dropped from 50 mls (milliliters) per minute at age 12 to barely 10 mls by age 30.

From 30 on, most of our body's functions lose about 1 percent of their original capacity per year. Depending on our personality and lifestyle, we begin to lose the resilience of youth. Smokers and others with self-destructive habits begin to slide rapidly downhill while those who adopt the Lifex Constants age more gracefully and slowly. In those who spent their youth acquiring a deep, bronze suntan, the skin's youthful elasticity disappears and is replaced by wrinkles.

Starting at 35, the statistical probability of dying doubles every eight years. By age 37 or so, the average person is halfway through life and a slow but inexorable decline begins. In sedentary people, the heart has difficulty speeding up to cope with increased physical exercise and our capacity to perform manual work begins to decline.

By age 40, the average man's height has shrunk by one-eighth to one-quarter inch and his hair has thinned. Both men and women of 40 begin to put on weight around the waist and chest. Lines appear in the face, and stamina and energy noticeably diminish.

The Third Stage of Life: Ages 40 to 60

After some thirty-five or more years of constant exposure to high-risk foods, inadequate exercise, punishing stress and cigarette smoke, the three neurophysical aging processes are well advanced. Most American males of 40 have arteries lined by cholesterol plaques. In both sexes, the immune system is often sluggish, and we are under stress for hours each day. It only takes a cluster of stressful life events—a divorce, loss of a loved one, unemployment, an investment setback—to create a level of stress sufficiently intense to trigger a degenerative disease.

During the Third Stage of Life, heart disease will strike one American male in five. After 50, women have an increasing risk of cancer of the breast and uterus. Gallstones, kidney stones, rheumatoid arthritis, varicose veins, hemorrhoids, diabetes and diverticulosis all become increasingly common. Although we contract a variety of diseases, the fact remains that almost all chronic diseases are caused by the same set of self-destructive habits.

The Decades Take Their Toll

A thick head of hair is often a harbinger of long life, a sign that cholesterol deposits have not choked off blood supplies to the scalp. However, production of the hormone androgen in the testes, which starts soon after puberty, also typically causes males to lose hair around the temples and in the center of the forehead, even in those destined for long life.

Between ages 20 and 50, the average man gains eleven pounds, his waist increases from 33 to 40 inches and his chest from 36 to 41 inches. Because lack of exercise leads to loss of bone and muscle, fat accumulation actually far exceeds the eleven pounds of weight gain. This is evidenced by a steady gain in the fat percentage of body weight, which while only 15 percent at age 20, gradually increases until by age 70, 30 percent of the average male body is fat.

High levels of estrogen production until menopause help women to preserve their feminine appearance and minimize accumulation of arterial cholesterol; but at age 50 or so, the ovaries reduce production of both estrogen and progesterone and women's tissues begin to lose their youthful resilience. Women who eat a high-fat diet and are chronically overweight begin menstruating earlier and enter menopause later in life than do lean women.

Their menstrual cycles have also been shorter. Through these circumstances, fat tissue in obese women continues to produce estrogen long after menopause and there is no longer much progesterone to counteract it. In this way, obese women are considered to have a higher rate of breast and uterine cancer than women of normal weight.

Between 50 and 65, overweight and sedentary men may also experience a mild male-menopause caused by a decrease in output of the male hormone testosterone. A decline in virility, stamina and strength gradually follows. In fit, healthy men who have adopted the Lifex Constants, the only effect of male menopause is a brief slowing in attaining erection and ejaculation.

By age 50, the average inactive adult is well advanced into middle age and the stage is set for a variety of chronic disease. Those below typically appear during the Third Stage of Life.

• **Stones: Kidney and Gallbladder**   Research from forty countries shows that a diet high in fats, animal protein and refined carbohydrates (sugar and white flour) increases risk of forming both kidney stones and gallstones. Conversely, a diet high in fiber and low in foods of animal origin lessens risk of stone formation.

Most urologists concur that kidney stones are formed from the uric acid in meat, which saturates the urine with calcium oxalate. When refined carbohydrates are eaten in addition, oversaturation occurs and precipitation of kidney stones begins. Strict vegetarians have a traditionally low rate of kidney-stone formation. One study in England, which compared fifty stone-prone persons with fifty healthy individuals, showed that all the healthy people ate a diet much higher in vegetable fiber.

Gallstones consist primarily of cholesterol produced by saturation of the bile when the diet is high in fat, meat and refined carbohydrates. A recent study at the University of Rome, Italy, on 160 gallstone patients found that all of the victims ate fewer fresh fruits and vegetables than an equal-sized control group of healthy persons. The authors of the study concluded that a low-fiber diet of animal-derived foods causes the body to produce an excess of deoxycholic acid, the precursor of gallstones.

Stones are, therefore, preventible by eliminating fat, meat and refined carbohydrates from the diet and replacing them with plenty of fresh fruits, vegetables, seeds and whole grains.

• **Cancer**   In 1971, the National Cancer Act precipitated a gigantic effort to overcome cancer. Gradually, as billions were spent fruitlessly trying to end cancer, it became increasingly apparent that cancer cannot be beaten or prevented by technology. Indeed, cancer rates are increasing, not falling.

More than one American in every four will get cancer during his or her lifetime. One in five will die of it. During 1982, 835,000 new cases of cancer were reported, 30,000 more than in 1981. Despite all the sophisticated technology, the chances of a person with cancer surviving for five years is still only two out of five.

While medical science has failed to win the war against cancer, several exciting scientific discoveries have recently emerged through which risk of cancer can be significantly lessened. It has been learned that cancer occurs in three distinct stages and that all three stage requirements must be met for cancer to develop. They are:

Stage 1. An initiator is first required to cause a mutation in the DNA of a cell. An initiated cell is benign and though it may lead to minor aberrations like aging spots, it retains a molecular structure that is recognized as self and friendly by the body's immune system. Among known initiators are all proven carcinogens including all chemicals toxic to the human body such as asbestos and petro-chemicals; high-frequency radiation such as ultraviolet sunlight and X-rays; tobacco and marijuana smoke; some food additives; nitrosamines in processed foods; aflatoxin; and excessive amounts of alcohol. Others like caffeine; foods that are salt-cured, salt-pickled or smoked; and hot dogs and bologna, are all strongly suspect. Implied as potentially carcinogenic because they are invariably toxic to human cells are all drugs, whether prescription, over-the-counter or "recreational." Some herbs could also be initiators.

Most people probably have several million initiated cells in their bodies. The number increases with age.

Stage 2. An activator is then required to transform an initiated cell to a malignant cell. It is believed that most activation is caused by fat, refined carbohydrates and animal protein in the diet, especially by polyunsaturated fats and hydrogenated vegetable oils. All fats also stimulate production of bile acids that are also activators.

A study of cancer mortality in forty countries by Dr. Gerhard N. Schrauzer found that breast and intestinal cancer are highest in countries with a high dietary intake of sugar, fat and meat, and lowest in countries where people eat more whole grains and fish. Population studies from dozens of other countries concur that wherever the diet is high in fat, cancer is more prevalent. Animal studies have also shown that whenever between 10 to 40 percent or more of daily calorie intake is derived from fats, incidence of cancer increases.

Still other studies have correlated cancers of the brain, nervous system and lymph system to a high intake of animal protein. All animal protein causes rapid growth and large body size, both of which increase cancer risk and also stimulate tumor growth. Such growth-producing foods as meat, dairy products, eggs and seafood have been linked to more than 50 percent of all male cancers and over 66 percent of female cancers. Most animal protein also has a high content of saturated fats. However, fish has a lower fat content, most of which is polyunsaturated. Low-fat dairy products are available in which most of the saturated fat has been removed. Yet all of these foods are still high in protein and capable of promoting rapid growth.

Fats of all types, including those found in both animal and marine life, have a proclivity for attracting and storing toxins such as pesticides and chlorinated hydrocarbons. The higher the fat content in any organism, the greater the residue of these potent carcinogens. Many fishes and seafoods are contaminated with residues of pesticides, herbicides and other agricultural chemicals that could initiate cancer.

Polyunsaturated fats are regarded as particularly dangerous because, even when refrigerated, they quickly become rancid on exposure to air. In just a day or two, freshly-pressed oils and vegetable fats can become heavily oxidized, a reaction which cannot be discerned by taste or appearance. When digested, these rancid oils release free radicals that swiftly activate initiated cells. Free radicals from oils are strongly suspect as tumor-producers in cancers of the breast, lung, upper esophagus, lymph glands and large intestine.

For years, Americans have been advised to switch from eating saturated fats to polyunsaturated fats to prevent atherosclerosis. Now we are finding that polyunsaturated fats activate more cancer than do saturated fats. Studies at both the Australian National University and the University of Western Ontario revealed that polyunsaturated fats induced more cancer in lab rats than did saturated fats. Strong indications are also emerging that polyunsaturated fats hasten the aging process.

Even more dangerous, as causes of both cancer and heart disease, are hydrogenated vegetable oils found in literally hundreds of commercially prepared food products from bread to margarine and mayonnaise.

Stage 3. Suppression of the Immune System. When a cell becomes activated, its molecular structure is so radically altered that its antigen is immediately recognized as non-self by patrolling lymphocytes. Swiftly, the body's immune system is alerted and the cell is destroyed. No one yet knows how many of our cells become activated daily but it appears probable that thousands of our cells become malignant every day. In older people who indulge in stimulants, take drugs, and eat a diet high in fat, meat and refined carbohydrates, the number could run into tens of thousands.

As long as our immune system remains strong and aggressive, no activated cell is likely to survive long enough to produce a tumor; however, when the immune system is suppressed by emotional stress, or by some prescription drug that interferes with the immune reaction, risk of cancer rises dramatically. Studies have shown that people who feel helpless and depressed, or whose self-esteem is eroded, frequently experience immune-system suppression and cancer often appears within a few months. The immune system can also become temporarily overloaded during an infectious disease and become unable to destroy malignant body cells.

Fat Identified As Cancer Risk

Once the steps in the cancer process had been identified, a thirteen-member scientific committee went to work under the aegis of the National Academy of Sciences. In 1982 they released a detailed report entitled *Diet, Nutrition and Cancer.* The report took the form of an analysis of all prior studies linking diet to cancer and was prepared by the Academy's National Research Council for the National Cancer Institute. Thus, it voiced the opinions of several of America's major scientific institutions and carried tremendous influence and prestige.

The report stated, in brief, that the average American derives 40 percent of his or her calories from dietary fat, mainly from red meats, butter, dairy foods, ice cream, poultry skin, cooking oils, hot dogs, hamburger and luncheon meats. The report went on to state "that of all dietary components studied, the evidence is most suggestive of a causal relationship between fat intake and the occurence of cancer." The committee recommended that Americans reduce their fat intake by at least one-fourth so that they derive no more than 30 percent of their calories from fat.

Although final proofs are not yet all in, literally hundreds of scientists, physicians and their families have drastically reduced intake of stimulants, drugs, high-risk foods and fats. Others have sought ways to attain emotional calm. Several doctors I talked with recently at a health conference had noted the committee's recommendation that not more than 30 percent of calorie intake should be from fats and that this was the upper limit, not the optimal amount. Several who had noticed that fat is implicated as a major cause in almost *every* degenerative disease felt that not more than 10 percent of daily calorie intake should be from fat. They believed that the National Academy of Sciences had recommended a conservative reduction from 40 to 30 percent in fat intake only because the Academy feared that the average American would not willingly accept any greater change in dietary habits.

The committee also reported that people who eat green leafy vegetables of the cabbage family; yellow vegetables and fruits; and seeds, tubers, beans, whole grains, potatoes, soybeans, chickpeas and other vegetables in place of animal fat and protein, have a far lower incidence of cancer of the lung, colon, rectum, gastro-intestinal tract, bladder, prostate, stomach and breast. The committee found evidence that replacing intake of animal foods with these and other vegetables inhibits the activity of cancer initiators and activators.

• **Type II Diabetes**   Deaths from diabetes increase rapidly for blacks after age 40 and for whites after 50. Approximately 10 percent of all diabetics have Type I insulin-dependent juvenile-onset diabetes mellitus. This appears early in life, may be hereditary, and requires insulin and a doctor's care. The remaining 90 percent of diabetes victims have Type II non-insulin dependent diabetes, a disease of middle life which we create ourselves through the vicissitudes of our own lifestyle.

Type II diabetes is caused by a diet high in fat and refined carbohydrates coupled with lack of physical exercise. Carbohydrates in food break down into glucose, a sugar which circulates in the bloodstream. Some of this glucose is stored in the liver and muscles as glycogen. Most is destined for storage in the body's fat cells. Before glucose can enter fat cells, insulin is required to transport it through the cell walls.

In response to rising glucose levels in the bloodstream, an area of the pancreas begins to manufacture insulin. Most Type II diabetics have plenty of insulin. The problem is that their fat cells are engorged with fat and the insulin receptors in these cells are unable to function. Thus the bloodstream remains filled with unused glucose and insulin. The excess insulin may damage artery walls and worsen atherosclerosis. Meanwhile, the excess glucose spills over into the urine, creating symptoms of diabetes.

If untreated, diabetes can lead to vision damage, numbness, skin and urinary infections, heart and kidney disease, gangrene, diabetic coma and even death.

People who are overweight, fail to exercise and overeat on a diet high in fats and refined carbohydrates, reduce the body's ability to metabolize excess glucose in the bloodstream. In fact, by age 50 their metabolic rate can drop 25 percent. If these habits are continued, the rate can decline an additional 25 percent by age 75. Because of the rapidity of this decline, almost half of all Americans over 50 show symptoms of diabetes when given a glucose tolerance test.

The condition is so widespread that doctors make allowances when interpreting glucose tolerance test readings in older people. Otherwise, half the population aged 50 or over would be diagnosed as diabetic. Although doctors bend test results to overlook millions of cases of borderline diabetes, the fact is that virtually everyone over 50 who is obese, who overeats on fats and refined carbohydrates, and who ignores the need for daily exercise, either has Type II diabetes or is a borderline case.

This is borne out by studies which show that 90 percent of all Type II diabetics are overweight, are high-fat eaters and do not exercise.

What may seem even more surprising is that Type II diabetes exists only for as long as we continue to indulge in these anti-life habits. When Type II diabetics change to a low-fat, high-fiber diet, and when they begin to exercise, by the time they have lost twenty pounds or so, their diabetes usually disappears. The records of cardiac rehabilitation and life extension centers are filled with thousands of case histories in which Type II diabetes disappeared in just three or four weeks after anti-life habits were replaced with Lifex Constants. The reversal is usually permanent for as long as the person continues to follow this upgraded lifestyle.

• **Rheumatoid Arthritis**   Recent research in immuno-therapy in cancer has uncovered a flood of new facts that clearly point to rheumatoid arthritis, and several associated articular dysfunctions, as being auto-immune diseases. Auto-immunity occurs when the immune system malfunctions and attacks the body's own cells instead of defending the body against invading bacteria.

Currently, some 6,500,000 Americans suffer from rheumatoid arthritis while other millions are victims of ankylosing spondylitis, systematic lupus erythematosus, scleroderma or similar connective tissue disorders. Rheumatoid arthritis, a systematic dysfunction, causes pain, swelling and inflammation in joints and typically strikes women aged 20 to 50. Anyone with rheumatoid arthritis or an associated articular dysfunction should see a doctor to ensure that damage will not result to eyes, kidneys or other organs.

Medical science has no cure for any type of arthritis. At best, it can only suppress painful symptoms by prescribing various anti-inflammatory drugs, some of which work by suppressing the immune system.

Many prominent allergists and immunologists now believe that rheumatoid arthritis, and possibly other types of auto-immune diseases, are basically caused by a diet high in fat, protein and refined carbohydrates. Smoking, lack of exercise, and a harmful response to stress all create a malfunction in the body's carbohydrate mechanism. One result is that the body develops an allergic sensitivity to foods to which we are addicted. Foods which many people often crave and eat frequently include alcohol and wine, sugar, refined wheat flour, dairy products, beef, caffeine, eggs, smoked and cured meats and fish, chocolate and soft drinks. (Drugs and nicotine are also common allergens as are chemicals, dust, pollen or animal danders.)

When these foods are eaten, a high blood-fat content causes the immune system to reject particles of an allergenic food. This triggers an immune response. The lymphocyte population begins to multiply and the white blood cell count soars. Swiftly, the bloodstream is filled with aggressive lymphocytes bent on destroying an invading infection.

But the only "enemy" is particles of food to which we are sensitive. Unable to find a real enemy, the armies of lymphocytes head for the most distressed tissue in the body. Through a process not fully understood, the extra stress of functioning as a joint cell somehow changes the antigen of cells in certain joints. Lymphocytes recognize these distressed cells as non-self.

Swiftly, killer lymphocytes spew lethal enzymes called "antigen-antibody complex" on to the already weakened joint cells. This poisonous combination eats away at cartilage, particularly in the knee, and suppresses production of synovial fluids which lubricate the joint.

The body responds to this attack by producing prostaglandins, which work to protect and heal the joint. They do so by creating heat, redness, inflammation and pain and by secreting large amounts of synovial fluid that cause the knee to swell. Phagocytes then move in to the joint, but large numbers are immediately poisoned by the antibody-antigen complex. As they die, the phagocytes release other powerful enzymes that further poison tissue cells.

The Body Itself Creates Arthritis

The pain, swelling, redness and inflammation of rheumatoid arthritis appear to be responses by the body to a condition caused by our self-destructive habits. Numerous studies have shown that when all fats, refined cabohydrates, junk food and most animal protein are removed from the diet, the victim recovers rapidly. Other programs obtain excellent results through using a five-day water fast.

Typical of such studies was one conducted by the Department of Medicine at Wayne State University, Michigan (reported in *Clinical Research*, Vol. 29, No. 4, 1981). The researchers found that rheumatoid arthritis symptoms were caused by fats in the standard American diet.

As long as the patients stayed on a diet low in fats, they remained free of symptoms. Two patients who exercised continual vigilance and avoided almost all sources of dietary fat for nine and fourteen months respectively, remained completely free of rheumatoid arthritis during these periods. Within forty-eight hours of eating a fatty meal, however, their symptoms returned.

Similar studies in England, Sweden, Japan, Israel and elsewhere have confirmed that the same anti-life habits that cause other degenerative diseases, also cause rheumatoid arthritis (and, most probably, other auto-immune diseases). When these destructive habits are replaced by Lifex Constants, rheumatoid arthritis soon disappears and remains in regression for as long as one continues to follow a healthy lifestyle.

Fat Shrinks Chances for Long Life

Obesity is frequently visible in Americans during the Third Stage in Life. Various studies have directly linked overweight with diabetes, hypertension, stroke, hernia, chronic nephritis and cirrhosis of the liver. It also heightens risk of cancer of the breast, uterus, liver and gallbladder. More specifically, two studies—made simultaneously by Dr. Artero Kesaniemi at the VA Medical Center, San Diego, and by Scott M. Grundy Ph.D., at the University of Texas Health Center, Dallas—both confirmed that obese persons have significantly higher LDL levels than persons of normal weight. A high LDL level is a significant risk factor for heart disease.

Dietary Fat Impairs Eyesight

During the Third Stage of Life, most Americans develop presbyopia, a rigidity in the eye lens caused as new cells overgrow the old. As the lens hardens, it becomes too large for the eye muscles to focus on close objects. To overcome this impairment, middle-aged people increasingly turn to bifocals and reading glasses.

Cholesterol from a diet high in animal fats is believed responsible for gradually restricting the amount of light reaching the retina. We begin to need brighter light to work by and we see less well in the dark.

More serious are cataracts, a cloudy patch over the lens which may require an operation to remove. Clinical studies have shown that cataracts are more common in people who are heavy consumers of milk and dairy products, or other dietary fats. Some opthalmologists have reported that when patients with beginning cataracts were placed on a low-fat diet, their condition improved or remained stable. Many were able to avoid a cataract operation.

The Fourth Stage of Life: Ages 60 to 80

From age 60 on, dramatic differences appear between those who continue high-risk habits and those who follow the Lifex Constants.

In men and women who eat the standard American diet, ignore the need for exercise, and who continue with other self-destructive habits, both mind and body steadily degenerate. By age 80, muscle strength is only 58 percent of what it was at 55. The ability to smell and taste diminishes. The number of taste buds and papilla decrease from 245 at age 30 to only 88 by age 70. To compensate, many older people crave increasing amounts of salt, sugar and condiments. The voice begins to quaver, especially in women, and hearing loses its sensitivity. Vision declines to 20/30 or less and we lose the ability to distinguish between blues and greens. Night vision deteriorates and peripheral vision weakens.

As the skin dries out, wrinkling increases. As cartilage grows, facial features increase in size. Between ages 30 and 70, the nose gains half an inch in length, the ears become longer and fatter, and the circumference of the head increases by approximately one inch.

Between 30 and 70, the average man loses one and one-eighth inches in height, due mostly to deterioration in the disks between spinal vertebrae. Years of flexing have worn down cartilage in joints and the synovial fluid that oils the joints is depleted. Most physicians assume that anyone over 60 have some degree of osteo-arthritis. Ligaments constrict, harden with age, and tear more easily.

Hair follicles become finer until by age 70, many people have hair as fine as a baby's. A combination of cholesterol deposits and hormones have caused balding to begin at the temples in men and the hairline may continue to recede until the entire head is bald. Hormone output, in fact, declines throughout the body. A diminished supply of epeniphrine reduces ability to respond to stress. As the body gradually loses ability to handle excess blood sugar, damage from alcohol and refined carbohydrates increases. Lymphocytes find it increasingly difficult to distinguish between self and non-self and incidence of auto-immune diseases grows steadily. Ability of nerve fibers to transmit signals slows, resulting in a decline in nerve reflex speed of 8 to 10 percent by age 70.

By 70, the kidneys can filter blood waste only half as efficiently as at age 35 and bladder capacity diminishes from two cupfuls to only one—leading older people to urinate more frequently. Between the same ages, the lungs lose so much elasticity that their capacity drops by 45 percent and the amount of oxygen entering the bloodstream is cut in half. This leads to thickening and stiffening of artery walls by extra tissue. As the blood vessels lose their elasticity, blood pressure rises.

During this stage in life, many men and women who eat a diet high in fats, animal protein and refined carbohydrates experience a painful outpouching of the colon walls called diverticulosis. As with most other degenerative diseases, diverticulosis is controlled when these foods are eliminated and replaced by a diet high in fresh, raw vegetables, fruits, seeds and in whole grains.

• **Benign Prostate Enlargement**   Need to urinate frequently is often associated in older men with enlargement of the prostate gland. The size of a walnut in youth, this horseshoe-shaped gland encloses the urinary tract at the base of the bladder. Any enlargement reduces the volume of the bladder and constricts the urinary tract. The gland is particularly sensitive to dietary intake of fat, animal protein, caffeine and alcohol. By age 65, most sedentary and overweight men have a prostate so enlarged that they must get up several times a night to urinate. In these same men, whose lifestyle supplies all three stage requirements for triggering cancer, the prostate is a common cancer site.

Most cases of prostate enlargement are benign, however, though the condition may become malignant later. The medical solution for benign enlargement is to either remove the gland entirely or to surgically pare it down to its original size. In the latter case, unless all self-destructive habits are controlled, the gland frequently becomes enlarged again.

Scattered around the country are some thirty-five small natural health resorts and nature cure spas which specialize in fasting and rejuvenation through lifestyle change. Over the years, almost every one of these institutions has completely reversed benign prostate enlargement in hundreds of men who have been willing to permanently replace their anti-life habits with Lifex Constants. Once a man's weight has returned to normal, a program of brisk daily exercise is established, and a diet built around intake of fresh fruits, vegetables, seeds and whole grains, the inflammation caused by years of undesirable habits gradually disappears and the prostate slowly returns to normal size.

• **Osteoporosis** Starting in the late 30s, both men and women begin to lose bone mineral. The loss accelerates in women after menopause, indicating a direct correlation with decline of estrogen production. From the late 40s on, the average woman loses between 8 and 10 percent of her bone density with each decade. Those who smoke, eat a diet high in animal protein, and ignore the need for abundant exercise, may lose bone calcium twice as rapidly. This condition contributes to the hip fractures that afflict 25 percent of elderly women. The hip bone is so thin, fragile and brittle that it shatters as they walk. Millions of other women 65 and over have bones so thin that the bones may break at the slightest blow.

Much of the calcium loss from bones has been traced to an imbalance in the calcium:phosphorus ratio resulting from a high intake of animal protein. Sheldon Margen, a nutritionist at the University of California, Berkeley, followed the histories of two thousand students since 1965 and found a straight-line relationship between loss of bone calcium and increased protein intake. Another Australian study found that meat-eating women frequently experienced a bone loss of 35 percent over a thirty-year period compared to only 18 percent for vegetarian women. Again, in 1979 a Department of Agriculture study found that a high protein intake caused a condition of osteoporosis in adult rats. Numerous studies have also shown that onset of osteoporosis is automatic in both sexes at any age whenever exercise is stopped for seven days or longer.

The medical solution is to prevent osteoporosis by prescribing estrogen for women after menopause. Study after study has shown, however, that osteoporosis can usually be prevented by diet, exercise and abstaining from smoking.

Several studies, including a recent research project at the University of Kentucky, have also demonstrated that, even in elderly women, bone lost through osteoporosis could be partially restored by exercising and increasing calcium intake.

Skim milk and low fat dairy products are high in calcium but both are also high in animal protein. In fact, 50 percent of the population has some degree of intolerance to lactose or milk sugar, causing an absorption problem. Many people aged 70 and over lose half their ability to absorb Vitamin D from sunlight. Vitamin D is essential for calcium absorption. As a result, physically active vegetarian women, who receive most of their calcium from green, leafy vegetables, have the best chance of preventing osteoporosis.

While some degree of bone loss is inevitable in women, osteoporosis is not a normal condition for older women. As thousands of healthy women centenarians have demonstrated, it is largely preventible through a lifestyle based on Lifex Constants.

Lifex Constants Are Good News

Those who opt for Lifex Constants between 60 and 80 frequently remain as strong, healthful and vigorous as between ages 40 and 60. During the Fourth Stage of Life, fit, healthy men and women continue to lead quality lives. Even as they approach 80, many still think in terms of new goals and career changes.

Mental Competence Can Increase Throughout Life

For example, recent studies have disproved earlier research which had concluded that, through losing 100,000 brain cells daily, memory and intelligence gradually decline. A study by Steven Zarit, Ph.D., a psychologist at the University of Southern California, revealed that a person's primary memory—the amount of information that can be held for processing at any given time—remains stable regardless of age. While some older people do experience a decline in ability to transform primary memory into long-term memory and then retrieve it, most older people are no more forgetful than when they were younger.

In another study at Pennsylvania State University by K. Warner Schaie, it was found that the majority of people at all ages studied retained their intellectual ability. In fact, those who remained mentally active were actually able to increase their mental competence, even into their nineties.

Senility, a term seldom used today by gerontologists, occurs in older people who are sick and infirm. As used today, senility is simply an umbrella term for twenty-five related diseases which cause changes in behavior and personality associated with aging. Most common is senile dementia of the Alzheimer type, a neurological disorder responsible for confusion and disorientation in about 1.5 million Americans. The majority of these people are in nursing homes.

Investigations have shown that the uncontrolled distribution of tranquilizers, sedatives and other drugs to quiet the elderly in nursing homes is responsible for approximately half of all cases of assumed senility in the elderly. When drug use has been stopped and the patients given exercise and care, many have recovered full use of their cognitive abilities. However, elderly people who have suffered a series of small strokes do experience lasting confusion and loss of memory.

Numerous studies have confirmed that healthy people retain intellectual and cognitive functions well into the ninth decade of life. Here again, older studies which reported a decline in oxygen glucose supply to the brain were based on samplings that included both healthy and infirm older people. The modern conclusion is that cerebral oxygen uptake and glucose levels do not decline in healthy older people until, at least, age 95.

More Aging Myths Exploded

Another myth recently exploded was the traditional belief that as we aged, the heart lost its ability to pump blood. A study presented in 1982 at the fifty-fifth session of the American Heart Association reported that researchers at Johns Hopkins University School of Medicine had shown that in fit, active people, the heart retains its ability to pump blood at full capacity throughout life. Prior studies had been made on an aging model that included both healthy and unhealthy older people.

Even though healthy older people may experience some loss in kidney function, they still have ample reserve to continue living in good health. They can function in good health on one-third of the original kidney capacity they had at age 30, on 20 percent of the thyroid substance, on 20 percent of the pancreas, and on 25 percent of the original liver capacity.

Nor do fit, healthy older people stop enjoying sex. Testosterone levels in men drop gradually to age 60 and then remain stable. Recent studies have confirmed that 80 percent of men remain sexually active through age 68, and 75 percent through age 78. Most find only that they need a longer recovery time before an erection and climax can be attained again.

The Fifth Stage of Life: Ages 80 to 100 Plus

Ninety-five percent of all Americans die between the ages of 77 and 93. Most who die before 85 are men.

Eighty is the threshold age past which few people who indulge to any extent in life-threatening habits manage to survive. For people who continue to eat high-risk foods, to smoke and to spurn regular exercise, homeostasis—the body's ability to maintain chemical balance—becomes increasingly difficult. Acid base, sugar level and body temperatures are easily thrown off balance by a large fatty meal, shoveling snow, or a few alcoholic drinks. Poor digestion, constipation, incontinence, trembling hands and diminished sight and hearing, all indicate that a person is losing the vitality needed to overcome life's challenges.

Age 85—The First Barrier Age

One reason why so few Americans live beyond 85 is that by that age, most people with a low HDL level have died. A high HDL level, which maintains the arteries free of cholesterol, must be maintained by regular daily exercise. HDL levels have been found elevated in all fit, healthy people over 80 and to remain elevated for as long as they choose to remain physically active.

So few people live beyond 85 that the standard abridged table of life expectancy stops at that age. Nonetheless, between 1966 and 1977 the mortality rate for people 85 and older dropped by 26 percent. A study at the University of Pennsylvania attributed this dramatic decline to the overall reduction in deaths from heart disease during the past two decades. During recent years, overall life expectancy in the United States has been increasing at an average rate of .33 years annually. It is felt this is due, primarily, to growing awareness of the risks of such high-risk habits as dietary fat, smoking and failing to exercise.

In 1983, life expectancy for a newborn American was seventy-four years (70 for men and 78 for women). Through elimination of childhood diseases, life expectancy at birth has almost doubled in the past century; however, for Americans 40 and over, the increase in life expectancy has been much less dramatic.

Through safer childbirth and by adopting Lifex Constants, more Americans are living longer. However, we are not reaching greater ages. The genetic upper limit of human life has hardly changed since ancient times. In classical Greece, people lived to approximately the same exceptional ages as today. Based on verifiable records, the *Guinness Book of Records* listed Mr. Shigechiyo Izumi of Japan, who died in 1981 at age 116, as the world's longest-lived man. In 1982, the world's longest-lived woman appeared to be Nancy Vine, a black American, then aged 117 and a resident of Cedar Hills Nursing Home in Jacksonville, Florida.

Although people live longer in sixteen other countries than in the United States, few centenarians anywhere live beyond 110. Based on careful records kept in Sweden, Canada, Britain and Ireland, only a handful of people reach 115. Several times each century, a few rare individuals may reach 117 or beyond.

These observations raised serious doubts concerning the actual number of authentic centenarians in the United States. During U.S. census counts, the ages of older persons are not verified and are often based on statements by relatives and friends. The 1970 U.S. Census listed 106,441 people as aged 100 or more. However, after two demographic statisticians used the Forward Survival Count and similar checks to analyze these figures, they estimated that not more than 4,800 Americans were actually aged 100 or over.

Age 93—The Second Barrier Age

Based on these new demographic models, a second barrier age occurs at 93, the average upper limit of life for long-lived women. Thus, we have a lifespan barrier at 85 for men and at 93 for women. Bear in mind, though, that these statistics are based on the average population of the United States.

For every American who extends his or her life through Lifex Constants, an estimated fifty shorten their lives through persisting with anti-life habits. Obviously, over the years, thousands of healthful centenarians have—either intentionally or by coincidence—successfully slowed their rate of biological aging. Their examples offer good reason to believe that by adopting positive personality and lifestyle characteristics, men and women can live for many active years beyond the barrier ages of 85 and 93.

5

Acquiring a Centenarian Personality and Lifestyle

Examine the life of any healthy, long-lived person and you will invariably discover that his or her personality and lifestyle reflect many of the Lifex Constants.

Victor Christen of Arcadia, California, is handsome, impeccably groomed, smartly dressed and ninety-four years old. Victor looks and acts like a youthful 60-year-old. He credits his vibrant health and vigor to his determination to stay physically and mentally active. Victor is both. He is reportedly still working full-time as one of the most successful salesmen at a large Chevrolet agency. Every day, he still drives thirty minutes each way to work and back.

Apart from being a widower and living alone, the life of Victor Christen is filled with health-building habits and attitudes. When interviewed, he told reporters that to live long, a person should eat in moderation and not smoke. Alcohol should be limited to one drink per day. He advised working at a steady but unhurried pace and to keep working for as long as possible. Through his work he is constantly meeting people and does not feel lonely or unneeded. He always has several goals, some for up to a year ahead, so that he constantly has something to look forward to.

Victor's comments reveal his perpetually youthful and optimistic personality. "Life is just beginning for me," he said. "I plan to live ten more years and then decide if I want to stay around for another ten."

Why do not more people think and act like Victor Christen? Why is it that for every American who adopts the Lifex Constants, fifty others continue to shorten their lives with unhealthy habits? Psychologists answer by pointing to our attitudes and personalities.

The Power of a "Type B" Personality

Some twenty years ago, San Francisco cardiologists Meyer Friedman and Ray Rosenman conducted a longitudinal study of 2,750 men in an attempt to relate personality characteristics to heart disease. Approximately 50 percent of the men were classified as Type A's: competitive, aggressive human dynamos obsessed with achievement. Forty percent were classified as Type B's: well-adjusted, relaxed men who cultivated calm, optimism and moderation. The remaining 10 percent fell in between.

During the following eight and one-half years, the Type A's showed an incidence of heart disease three times greater than the Type B's. When a heart attack did occur, it proved fatal twice as often for Type A's as for Type B's. Thus, a straight-line correlation was confirmed between Type A personality and heart disease.

Since then, psychologists have identified a cancer-prone Type C personality.

Researchers have found a dramatic difference in health and longevity between persons with a Type A or C personality and those with a Type B. People with Type A or C personalities have negative attitudes toward health and are content to practice a minimum of good health habits. Their negative attitude toward health and aging frequently becomes a self-fulfilling prophecy. The belief that life expectancy is three score years and ten is a typical self-fulfilling prophecy that shortens millions of lives unnecessarily. "Eat, drink and be merry for tomorrow we may die," is another self-fulfilling prophecy that frequently leads Type A and C personalities to believe they will be over the hill by 40, middle-aged by 50, and retired on a disability pension a few years later. As Marilyn Ferguson wrote in *The Aquarian Conspiracy* (J.P. Tarcher, 1980), "Of all the self-fulfilling prophecies in our culture, the assumption that aging means decline and poor health is probably the deadliest."

Healthy, Long-Lived People Have Disease-Resistant Personalities

With few exceptions, every fit and healthy long-lived person has a Type B personality. This desirable mindset, known to psychologists as an "integrated" or "disease-resistant" personality, is a pre-requisite for anyone seeking optimal health and long life. The fact that you are reading this book may indicate that you are already a Type B. Even if you are an unmistakable Type A or C, however, you do not have to remain one. Thousands of Americans have successfully modified their Type A or C personality traits into a Type B, often with dramatic results.

For example, studies involving thousands of initially healthy people with Type-A personality traits have confirmed that having this personality doubles or triples the risk of heart disease. Yet in a later study at Stanford University, funded by the National Heart, Lung and Blood Institute, it was found that people with Type A personalities who modified their Type A characteristics, particularly those of anger and hostility, had fewer than half the expected number of heart attacks. This study provided abundant evidence that changing your personality can change your life.

The first step in such a transformation is to have a clear idea of exactly what constitutes a Type A or C personality and how they contrast with a Type B profile.

Type-A Archetypal Traits

The classical Type A person is a dynamic, high achiever who seeks power and influence through upward mobility. (Males outnumber female Type A's by at least two to one.) Type A's are frequently intense, extroverted, impatient and uncompromising workaholics who schedule more and more projects into less and less time. They find it stressful to relax and feel guilty when not working.

The Type A personality stems from a feeling of insufficiency and lacking. So they work feverishly to secure more money and possessions, more approval, a prestigious career, and high living, all in the belief that by achieving all these things they will find happiness.

Until they get what it is they think they need, Type A's feel inferior and disappointed. When they achieve something, they may experience brief satisfaction because, for the moment, they stop desiring something else. But soon, they may become fearful and anxious of losing what they had just achieved. So their happiness and contentment evaporates. They believe that only by achieving something else can they become happy once more. So off they go at a furious pace once again. Eventually, the whole cycle is repeated. As they seek yet another goal, Type A's become compulsively driven. This frantic pace destroys the very ease and contentment through which happiness is attained.

A frenetic pace becomes the core of a Type A person's life. Their entire lives are soon programmed by rigid, self-imposed deadlines, which create a frantic sense of urgency and a compulsive fear that time is running out. This exaggerated response to time triggers the Fight or Flight reaction so that it never shuts off completely. Type A's live in a continuous state of emergency that speeds up all their body rhythms and physiological functions, which creates high blood pressure, high rates of heartbeat, respiration and hormone production, and constant muscle tension. These stresses suppress the immune system and may lead to illness. Stress may lead to hypertension and platelet clumping and even stroke.

These hazardous symptoms are less evident in Type A women, but studies have demonstrated that many women with heart disease have Type A personalities. To pacify their stress, many Type A's of both sexes may become heavy smokers or indulge in other stimulants or drugs. Their lifestyle causes Type A individuals to become highly irritated with inefficiency or delay. To save time, they regularly do several things at once, like eating and driving, or breakfasting and shaving. Type A's operate under such intense time pressure that any unforeseen contingency can create an emotional explosion.

If you see yourself in this pattern, the following symptoms may help to confirm a Type-A personality trend. Having an insatiable need to know and collect information about your work; quantifying everything in numbers, including your own and others' achievements; losing all interest in nature and things of art and beauty; playing every game to win, even with children; frequent use of pronouns, "I, me, my and mine." (A study by Dr. Larry Scherwitz revealed that the more a cardiac patient uses these words, the more severe are his or her heart disease symptoms.)

Above all, hostility is the key trait that identifies all Type A's. They are often angry people who feel that the world around them is threatening and unfriendly. So hazardous to health are these characteristics that approximately 70 percent of all Type A persons die before reaching age 65.

Type-C Archetypal Traits

Type C persons tend to suffer quietly and internally. They spend much time serving others who may take advantage of them. Type C's are private people who stifle their emotions. They become tense and unable to express their feelings or to release anger and other negative emotions. Instead, their internalized stress works directly through the central nervous system to suppress the immune system. Stress may manifest as an ulcer, ulcerative colitis, gallstones, gastritis or chronic constipation and diarrhea.

Stress may even cause the immune system to malfunction and set off auto-immunity. Type C's undergo tremendous inner conflict by pretending to appear outwardly calm while inwardly they are worried and anxious. Their attitude prevents them from becoming truthful and open. Thus, Type C's have difficulty developing or maintaining close relationships. Should a close relationship fail, many Type C's are so discouraged that, having experienced disappointment once, they give up hope and never try again. Some may be so dependent that they refuse to be separated or divorced. They seek affection yet reject it when offered. Lack of self-esteem makes many Type C's feel powerless, unworthy, rejected, cynical and despairing.

This attitude leads confirmed Type C's to become unwell and significantly increases their risk of cancer and diabetes. Being unwell may also get them the sympathy and attention that they did not receive when well. When sickness earns such rewards, it destroys all incentive to become well again.

In the decline into Type C depression, there exists a point beyond which people become powerless to help themselves. They feel it is hopeless to try to improve their personality or habits. At this stage, a Type C needs professional help.

Fortunately, the majority of Type C people have much milder symptoms. The realization that one is clearly a Type C, is sufficient motivation to cause the average person to want to turn his or her health habits around.

Type-B Archetypal Traits

Most Type B people have learned to respond to stress in positive ways. They are willing to accept what they cannot change. Many Type B people actively welcome change; thus, a Type B person is in full control of his or her life and health. They also feel in full control of their environment and of sources of stress, including job, money and family. They work hard and often accomplish much, but they are unwilling to build their lives around their careers. They do not strive for upward mobility nor do they take their work problems home.

Type B people have many goals but few deadlines. They invariably have a purpose in life and are active, but they live at a relaxed pace and are liberated from time-pressure stress.

Type B's are well-adjusted, confident people with high self-esteem and a strong self-image. They are free of aggression or hostility and see no reason to display their ego or their achievements. Type B's can relax without guilt and their leisure is devoted to fun rather than competition. A Type B seldom has the need to smoke, to drink to excess or to take drugs. Many have instituted the Lifex Constants. Type B's seldom become sick. Even if a catastrophe occurs, they possess the resilience to bounce back and begin again. Except for obvious cases requiring a diagnosis or emergency treatment, they studiously avoid all dependence on doctors, medications, hospitals and surgery.

Type B's obtain an abundance of social support from a strong network of relatives and friends. Most feel close to their parents. The typical Type B person experiences a strong feeling of love for other people. They are invariably calm and serene, optimistic, and content. Their ability to remain calm while the world around them may be in chaos permits them to effectively handle crisis or emergency. This same ability allows them to enjoy the adventure of sampling new experiences and of taking prudent risks.

Above all, Type B's have a refreshing sense of aliveness. They are willing to become involved with a cause, a purpose, a goal, and to make a contribution. They have not deserted their ideals. Type B's retain a strong sense of courage and optimism because they have confidence that no matter what the future brings, everything will turn out all right. They enjoy spontaneous, unplanned activities and they retain a youthful curiosity for life. This helps them to concentrate on the good things in their lives and not the bad. While they do have concern for the future, they live in and enjoy the present moment to the fullest.

Finally, Type B people care for their bodies. They lead a well-paced life that includes time for exercise and recreation and they take care not to over-indulge in food and drink.

These Type B traits are common to every healthful centenarian. Long-lived cultures, such as the Seventh Day Adventists and the Mormons consist of predominently Type B personalities. As described in Chapter 1, these groups outlive the general population by seven to eleven years.

Breakthrough into a Centenarian Personality

The closer you can come to having a Type B personality, the greater the likelihood that you will live a long, healthy and active life, consequently, the first step is to transform yourself from being a Type A or C, or a mild Type B, into a strong and unmistakable Type B personality.

Most of us are aware of which personality type we lean toward most. If we recognize ourselves as predominantly a Type A or C, we should concentrate on changing our basic personality configuration to that of a Type B. Personality is not irrevocable. Even if we recognize our personality as only mildly Type B, we can strengthen this trend by adopting more Type B traits.

Many long-lived people have made personality switches at some point in their lives. Many have made mid-life career changes. Others simplified their lives and slowed their pace of living. Even late in life, people have shed their self-destructive habits and transformed themselves into long-lived Type B personalities.

Source of Long Life: The Type B Personality

Identification of the Type B personality by Friedman and Rosenman was soon followed by a variety of other studies, all of which unmistakably linked Type B behavior with high-level wellness and long life. A Gallup poll of nonegarians identified exactly the same Type B patterns in longevous people.

A survey of long-lived Americans by the Center for the Study of Aging and Human Development at Duke University also found that attitude played a vital role in being long-lived. Those who lived longest had the strongest positive thoughts. They remained physically, mentally and socially active throughout life. When faced with adversity, they refused to give in. In short, their personalities included many of the traits associated with Type B's.

Studies with similar conclusions are legion. A survey of 480 elderly California readers of *Prevention* Magazine by Linus Pauling, Ph.D., and James E. Enstrom observed that these men and women practiced many good health habits such as not smoking, eating little meat or salt, refraining from eating white flour and sugar, and taking vitamin and mineral supplements. Compared to the general population of the United States, their death rate was 32 percent lower; and for the women in the study, the death rate was 46 percent below that of the general population. The key factor, it turned out, was not any specific habit but their overall positive attitude to life and health.

A similar study in Wales (reported in the *American Journal of Clinical Nutrition*, November, 1982) compared a group of health-minded vegetarians with a similar group of health-minded non-vegetarians. Results showed that the vegetarians had a significantly lower risk of heart disease. But the researchers also found that, during the period of the study, the age-adjusted death rate among both vegetarians *and* meat eaters was half that of the general population. The researchers concluded that, regardless of diet, the real motivating force behind the reduced mortality rate was a strong health-conscious attitude and personality.

In contrast, the Gallup poll and other studies have confirmed that people who strive and compete, or who display hurried, hostile behavior, are all at considerable risk for heart disease.

The changeover to a Type B personality reduces the devastating effects of being a Type A or C. As soon as time-pressure urgency is controlled, most Fight or Flight symptoms disappear. Blood cholesterol levels drop as well as blood pressure, heartbeat and respiratory levels.

Equally positive results follow when negative Type C thinking is changed to a more positive Type B attitude. This was confirmed in a 1983 study by Dr. David McClelland, a Harvard psychologist, who tested the immune defense reaction in one hundred volunteers after showing them movies depicting love, humor and compassion and then a film depicting violence and hate. Results showed that positive emotions such as humor, love and compassion boosted resistance to disease while negative emotions suppressed the immune system. Other studies have shown that cancer often worsens soon after diagnosis, indicating that the shock of learning that one has cancer creates negative emotions that also suppress the immune system. All of these studies suggest a significantly reduced risk of disease through changing from a Type C to a Type B personality.

How to Turn Your Personality Around

Several million Americans are already committed to changing their personalities and lifestyles in deference to a longer, healthier life.

Aging involves every function in the body and mind. No single technique can make us long-lived; however, a change in personal philosophy does motivate us into adopting a lifestyle based on the Lifex Constants. This is called the Wellness Lifestyle. A Type B personality coupled with the Wellness Lifestyle form a matrix to extend our lives by many years.

Our personality is merely a subtle complex of beliefs, thoughts and values about ourselves and the world around us. Our lifestyle becomes an extension of our personality. Hence, once we acquire the Type B personality, the Wellness Lifestyle automatically follows.

Unfortunately, there seems to be no dynamic technique by which we can make a sudden and total personality switch. Instead, many psychologists suggest that we need to begin with a sincere desire to be healthy and long-lived. Merely being aware of the risks involved in remaining a Type A or C motivates most people to take the necessary steps to build a Type B personality.

However, the Lifex Constants are powerful tools for positive change. We can help end the suffering of being a Type A, or the helplessness of being a Type C, by taking the following transformational steps. You may find it easier to work on one aspect at a time rather than to try to change everything immediately.

• **Slow down and liberate yourself from all time schedule pressure.** Reduce the pace of your life so that you move, eat, work, play, talk, think and drive at a leisurely pace. Reschedule your life to eliminate any non-essential activities that can create pressure or increase demands on your time. Allow ample time for frequent relaxation and for fun, games and vacations with your family. Be assertive in turning down all unwanted responsibilities.

• **Expect optimal wellness and longevity as a normal condition of life.** Acquire a positive attitude about health and aging. Consider sickness and death before age 85 to be unusual.

• **Assume complete control of your life. You have the power to make changes. Accept full responsibility for your own health and well-being.** Accept what you cannot change and stop worrying about it. In particular, learn the uselessness of adopting a passive role toward health by assuming you can depend on medication or surgery to make you well while you continue to indulge in health-destroying habits.

• **Welcome change and adventure.** Each day, make a small change in your life. Consider walking or driving to work by a new route. Spend an evening doing something you have never done before. Become mildly venturesome. Learn to react positively to changes by becoming flexible and adaptable. Becoming open to change makes us far less vulnerable to stress. Transforming our personalities becomes much less stressful when we become willing to explore unfamiliar habits and new ways of living.

• **Assess your direction and goals.** If you were to live your life over again, would you still be doing the same thing? Look at your position and situation as a result of being a Type A or C. Consider where you would prefer to be going as a Type B. Make an assessment of goals and purposes for your new Type B life that would enhance your health and life expectancy. Make an inventory of the choices, options and priorities available.

• **Have a sense of humor.** Life is not serious. Try to see the fun side and humor in everything. Have a hearty laugh as often as possible, even if it is at yourself. Make others laugh if you can.

• **Eliminate aggressive upward mobility.** Compete with yourself instead of with others. Try to beat your own records and standards of achievement.

• **Remain involved but relaxed.** Without creating time pressures, stay involved in a cause, hobby or anything that interests you. Only by continuing to make a contribution can you have the support of a network of friends.

These steps can get you started. Others will occur as you review the list of Type-B archetypal traits and as you read about each Lifex Constant in the remainder of this book.

Adopting the Wellness Lifestyle

Personality and lifestyle are so interwoven that the moment you begin to adopt a Type B Personality, you also begin to work into the Wellness way of life. The Wellness Lifestyle represents a healthy balance between the various Lifex Constants. It does not mean having to give up everything that is good or enjoyable.

Not long ago, a newspaper article stated that science had discovered how we can stay healthier and extend our lives by adopting the Lifex Constants. "But you won't like it," the writer said, "it means giving up almost everything."

"Which do you really want?" the writer concluded. "The good life or a longer life?"

The writer was saying that he and others prefer to risk premature death rather than relinquish destructive habits. That the majority of Americans still prefer the dubious pleasures associated with harmful habits is indicated by records showing that only 6 percent of all adults really enjoys true health.

Despite these irrational yet persistant beliefs, many thinking people are beginning to realize that the Wellness Lifestyle *is* the good life. In contrast to the pain and suffering that eventually strikes everyone with self-destructive habits, the Wellness Lifestyle offers an immediate improvement in health and well-being followed by a full lifetime of healthful fun and contentment.

Changing Lifestyle to Lengthen Life

All it takes to begin living the Wellness way is to adopt as many Lifex Constants as you can conveniently work into your lifestyle. Some Constants, such as diet and exercise, are things you can change as soon as you are ready. Still others, such as eliminating health hazards from your life, such as tobacco or unnecessary drugs, should be given immediate priority. Others, like boosting your will to live or changing your response to stress, may require more time.

Which Constants you decide to work on first and which you decide to leave until later will depend on your own personal values, priorities and circumstances. But here, as a general guide, is a list of all the Constants in the order in which you might consider adopting them into your lifestyle.

Lifex Constant   2. Refrain from Smoking and Using Other Harmful Stimulants

Lifex Constant   3. Follow Sound Nutritional Practices

Lifex Constant   4. Eat Sparingly

Lifex Constant   5. Exercise Regularly

Lifex Constant   9. Maintain an Erect Posture

Lifex Constant   1. Minimize Dependence on Medical Care

Lifex Constant 16. Practice Moderation

Lifex Constant   6. Mobilize a Store of Physical Energy

Lifex Constant   7. Avoid Becoming Tired or Fatigued

Lifex Constant 15. Develop Sound Sleep Habits

Lifex Constant   8. Maintain Recommended Body Weight

Lifex Constant 23. Keep Growing Intellectually

Lifex Constant 14. Consider Yourself As Old As You Feel

Lifex Constant 27. Make Clear, Bold, and Unequivocal Choices

Lifex Constant 11. Adopt a Flexible Attitude and Accept Necessary Change

Lifex Constant 19. Cultivate a Loving, Friendly Attitude

Lifex Constant 22. Work at Something Meaningful and Challenging Throughout Life

Lifex Constant 24. Seek Maximum Independence

Lifex Constant 18. Develop a Powerful Will to Live

Lifex Constant 12. Cultivate an Optimistic Outlook

Lifex Constant 13. Slow Down. Avoid Stress. Live in the Present Moment

Lifex Constant 25. Be Ready to Take Prudent Risks

Lifex Constant 20. Develop a Supportive Network of Friends and Relatives

Lifex Constant 17. Develop a Sense of Humor and Cultivate Spontaneity

Lifex Constant 21. Enjoy Regular Sexual Activity

Lifex Constant 26. Have Faith in Something Spiritual

Lifex Constant 10. Live in a Healthy Environment

Readily attainable constants are such habits as exercise and nutrition that we can choose to make part of our lives almost immediately. As we begin to practice these habits, and notice immediate improvement in our health, it encourages us to work on the more personal psycho-social Constants. These Constants, which often take longer to bring about, improve the quality of our emotions and relationships.

Of all the Constants, work fulfillment (Lifex Constant 22) has a greater impact on health and longevity than any other single influence. However, each of the Constants works synergistically with all others so that the overall benefit of half a dozen Constants is several times greater than the sum of the benefits of each Constant considered separately. The benefits of exercise, for instance, are doubled when exercise is practiced in conjunction with a low-fat diet. In this way, each Constant interacts with all others to form a holistic life extension program through which we can attain exceptional health and longevity.

Planning Your Personal Odyssey for Long Life

By working your way down the list, you can build a common sense lifestyle that balances sound nutrition with exercise, work with play, and regularity of life with spontaneous fun and adventure. Since each Constant reinforces the benefits of all other constants in your life, you would soon find yourself empowered with surprisingly high levels of energy and health.

If seven simple good health habits such as those in the California Department of Health study (see Chapter 1) can extend life by eleven and one-half years, consider the potential of a program that includes *every* factor known to extend human life. Instead of a mere seven simple habits, you can have twenty-seven powerful Constants all working together to restore your health and prolong your life.

The following chapters describe how to put each Lifex Constant into practice. Each chapter also contains information on life extension and will add to your understanding of aging and health.

With this information you will be ready to decide the order in which to adopt each Constant into your own life extension program. Naturally, it could take several years to achieve such Constants as having a satisfying work situation, or to move from a large, stressful city to a safe, restful environment. Indeed, some Constants may not appear to be for you at all at this time.

Yet, most of us can begin to extend our lives immediately by incorporating as many Constants into our lifestyle as we conveniently can.

As Dr. Ira H. Cisin, a member of the California Department of Health research team, summed it up, "Good health practices take work and self-discipline and they can be inconvenient. But the pay-off is tremendous in terms of a healthier and longer life."

6

The Holistic Approach
to Life Extension

"I don't take medicine of any kind. I don't know that I'd want to live if I had to be doctored all the time. I've never been sick to amount to anything." These words, spoken by Mrs. Anna Le May of Memphis, Tennessee, on the occasion of her 102 birthday some years ago, exemplify the attitude that many healthy centenarians have toward avoiding medical treatment.

Being circumspect about medical care is a Lifex Constant that occurs repeatedly in the profiles of many healthy, longevous people. William Pownall of Boynton Beach, Florida, who celebrated his 101 birthday in 1973, cited minimizing medical care as the key health-building habit in his long, active life. He was 85 when he first visited a doctor.

As equally determined to avoid unnecessary medical care was David Trumble. In 1982, at the age of 114, Trumble was Canada's oldest citizen. All his life he had worked tirelessly as a logger and farmer until he retired at age 96. Trumble would probably have never visited a doctor at all had he not broken his back in a logging accident when he was 75. At the hospital, he was told he would never walk again. But David Trumble, like so many centenarians, possessed such resources of stamina and resilience that he was able to rebound and recover. At 114, he was still walking eight miles every day and he continued to dance several evenings each week.

LIFEX CONSTANT 1: Minimize Dependence on Medical Care

Longevous people lessen contact with doctors, hospitals, drugs and surgery.

A Type-B personality trait that is common to many long-lived people is their willingness to assume responsibility for their own wellness and to play an active role in taking charge of their own health.

By comparison, many people depend on drugs and medical technology when they become ill. This passive attitude identifies a predominently Type A or C personality.

This passivity, which is strongly supported by the pathology-management industrial complex (composed of physicians, hospitals, and pharmaceutical manufacturers) continues to dominate the thinking of our culture. The public is still largely conditioned to the belief that health depends primarily on intervention by a physician and that the sooner a disease is discovered and diagnosed, the sooner drugs and surgery can cure it. This widespread attitude creates a non-supportive environment that destroys our intentions to take care of our health. Accepting responsibility for our health is completely contrary to the popular beliefs that pervade our culture.

Runaway Medical Costs

Medical costs have skyrocketted to such heights that many people under 65 cannot afford to become sick.

Even though 75 percent of Americans are covered by some form of health insurance, authorities recognize that possession of health coverage inhibits incentive to pursue a wellness lifestyle. Surveys show that insured persons consult a physician twice as often as those who are not insured.

Before choosing to rely on medical care to stay well, we should become aware of the sweeping changes that are transforming the entire pathology management business. The familiar family practitioner and the non-profit community hospital are rapidly disappearing. Hospitals are being taken over by large chains, some of which are run by powerful profit-making corporations.

The hospital industry is already too large, having too many beds. To stay in business, neighboring hospitals must duplicate expensive equipment and compete for patients. As chain hospitals offer services that compete with physicians, doctors are being forced into group practice where they can profit from auxiliary services like labs and diagnostic equipment. In the process, doctors are being transformed into physician-businesspeople. Both hospitals and physicians are being forced to aggressively market their services in order to survive.

To keep profits rolling in, some hospital administrators are reported to be putting subtle pressure on physicians to order more lab tests and diagnostic procedures and to produce more admissions. This increases the risk that your doctor may recommend an unnecessary operation or some other form of unnecessary treatment.

In an article entitled *The Great Pacemaker Scandal* in its October 1983 issue, *Reader's Digest* reported that at least 200,000 cardiac pacemakers had been unnecessarily implanted in older Americans. The article stated that some doctors in the United States have taken bribes and kickbacks from pacemaker manufacturers.

Other doctors push and sell expensive procedures rather than teach their patients economical ways to lessen dependence on medical care. Most doctors are aware that alternative therapies are often more effective in reversing degenerative diseases than are drugs. They find it much easier and more profitable, however, to write a prescription than to spend an hour trying to convince a patient to eliminate self-destructive habits. Thus medical advice today is hardly impartial.

Meanwhile, patients themselves are demanding drugs to relieve many ailments and inconveniences. Thousands of drugs are available not only to combat disease but to prevent conception, to lose weight and to offset many social inconveniences.

Investment magazines feature articles on how to profit from the growing health care boom by purchasing stocks in drug companies and hospital management chains. Medical care and drugs today are designed primarily to yield large profits for physicians, hospitals and pharmaceutical manufacturers.

To safeguard their profits, the pathology management industry has created a legal and political hold on many aspects of the health care field. Chiropractors and naturopaths are barely tolerated and forms of alternative therapy are viewed with skepticism. Many doctors discourage patients from turning to sources of alternative therapies, such as cardiac rehabilitation centers; these sources siphon off income and expose medical treatment as unnecessary.

Lost Dimensions in Healing

In many cases, the warm, human touch of the family doctor has been replaced by an impersonal attitude, a sterile production line treatment, and by quantifying lab tests. In fact, lab tests are surprisingly inaccurate. A study made in 1983 at the Houston, Texas, VA Hospital found that young doctors often make significant diagnosis errors, or miss important symptoms, in almost 66 percent of their cases. A similar study at a Harvard teaching hospital showed the same rate of diagnosis error among more experienced doctors.

In both cases, the oversights were due to reliance on technology and machines instead of the traditional physical exam and a careful history check.

Through such diagnostic errors, millions of Americans have had unnecessary operations. Other untold millions have been unnecessarily placed on maintenance drugs with such adverse reactions as impotence, headaches, skin rashes, nausea and suppression of the immune system.

Antibiotics have been so overprescribed that hospitals in the United States have become fertile sources of hepatitis and infections. Iatrogenic diseases— consisting primarily of complications from surgery, adverse drug reactions and trauma—now rank as the eleventh cause of death in America. Studies have shown that up to 25 percent of all people who enter hospitals contract an iatrogenic disease they did not have when admitted.

As a result, approximately 15 to 20 percent of all medical procedures are done to safeguard doctors against malpractice suits, including unnecessary exposure to X-rays.

The Problem with Medication

Many drugs produce adverse side effects, but many drugs also fail to work. So extensive is the list of ineffective drugs that a national consumer organization, Public Citizen, has published a book entitled *Pills That Don't Work*. It describes 610 prescription drugs that lack evidence of effectiveness. Several other books have been published entirely devoted to the risks and side effects of prescription drugs. In 1983, the FDA concluded an eleven-year study of 700 popular non-prescription drugs. Two-thirds of the drugs studied were found ineffective and approximately half of these were also found to be unsafe.

Obviously, many medical procedures for conditions such as hemorrhoids, varicose veins or damaged knee cartilage offer great benefit and little risk. Equally obvious, however, is that when it comes to degenerative diseases, many treatments consist of powerful drugs and procedures for persons who are unwilling or unable to help themselves. Medical treatments for cancer, heart disease, hypertension, rheumatoid arthritis, diabetes, kidney, and similar problems have the potential to cause extensive harm.

Search for Alternatives

As medical science turns increasingly away from traditional humanistic healing practices toward biochemical, technological and pharmaceutical developments, a growing alienation is developing between the public and the pathology-management industrial complex. As one medical scandal after another is exposed, a credibility gap is growing between people and their doctors.

Millions of Americans have already lost confidence in the medical profession and are looking in new directions. They are rediscovering the lost dimensions of healing in the holistic health and healing movement. Through embracing a series of gentle, non-invasive therapies, the holistic movement has restored love and caring as essential qualities in all forms of healing.

The holistic approach to healing is not something that can be delivered on request. It represents the belief that emotional stress is transformed by the mind into physiological disease. Our ease is thus transformed into *dis-ease.* It therefore follows that through self care, we can learn to restore our ease and, in the process, overcome most forms of dysfunction.

For this to happen, we must use a Whole Person (holistic) approach based on the physical, mental, emotional and spiritual aspects of health and healing.

In place of a battery of diagnostic tests, a holistic practitioner is more likely to ask how your job, family and money problems may be affecting your health. Instead of recommending severe medication or surgery for heart disease, a holistic practitioner might suggest exercise and nutrition, deep relaxation, guided imagery and meditation—natural therapies which function on the physical, emotional, mental and spiritual levels. The holistic approach assumes that every disease is a problem of the general health of the Whole Person.

This is in direct contradiction to the methodology of orthodox medicine, which has spent the last hundred years separating the mind from the body and then decompartmentalizing both into scores of specialties. The holistic approach puts them back together to form a single Whole Person mind-body continuum. Holistic practitioners, in fact, are now using a bio-psychosocial model of the Whole Person in which our psychological states and our degree of adjustment to society are given equal ranking with the physical body in determining overall health.

Backlash Against Crisis Medicine

The holistic approach to health embraces every type of therapy with demonstratable healing value. This naturally includes orthodox medical treatment. Whenever medical care can do most good, the holistic movement strongly endorses it. Holistic health aims to complement medical care, not to challenge it. For any type of injury, emergency, trauma or other crisis, modern medicine has few substitutes. This book is not intended to discourage use of orthodox medical care whenever it is clearly needed.

Problems arise because medical science tends to over-react with crisis treatment for slow-onset degenerative diseases.

The inadequacies of mainstream medicine become apparent when we recall that many degenerative diseases are caused by our own destructive habits. A major principle of holistic healing is that when the cause of disease is removed, the body becomes a self-healing entity. When we stop punishing our bodies with self-destructive habits and replace them with healthful Lifex Constants, most degenerative diseases will gradually disappear. Only where damage is irrepairable, as with cancer or emphysema, are degenerative diseases non-reversible.

The Results of Anti-Life Habits

Drugs and surgery cannot cure negative habits. Doctors cannot eat for us, exercise for us, or stop smoking for us. Instead of removing the cause of degenerative diseases, doctors can only alleviate symptoms like stiffness or pain. By-pass operations do not remove the cause of heart disease. Only we can remove the cause of degenerative disease by replacing our health-destroying habits with Lifex Constants.

Most Diseases Can Be Prevented

Most degenerative diseases can be prevented and the majority can be controlled and perhaps reversed by harmless, natural therapies such as exercise, diet and stress management.

A large number of studies have demonstrated, for example, that athero-sclerosis can be controlled by exercise, a low-fat diet and stress management. These Constants can control coronary artery disease, angina, hypertension, Type II diabetes, obesity, and other ills. Without using drugs, cardiac rehabilitation centers have repeatedly lowered cholesterol levels in large groups of people and beneficial changes have followed, including gradual reversal of artery damage. Tens of thousands of Americans have given themselves revitalized coronary arteries by a holistic approach based on diet, exercise and emotional calm.

A typical example is the case of Eulah Weaver who, at the age of 81, was suffering from congestive heart failure, coronary artery damage, high blood pressure, liver trouble and crippling arthritis. She signed up as a volunteer to test the cardiac rehabilitation program then being developed at the original Pritikin longevity center. She commenced a program of gradually increased daily exercise. She began a diet composed 80 percent of vegetables, fruits and grains, 10 percent of protein and 10 percent of fat.

One by one, Mrs. Weaver's symptoms gradually eased. Within months, she had more energy and was jogging one and a half miles every day. Four years after she began the program as an invalid, Eulah Weaver finished the 1,500 meter run in the Senior Olympics, winning a gold medal and breaking the record for women in her age group. In 1979, at age 90, Eulah Weaver was still actively jogging and pedalling her way to fitness. She had stayed faithfully with her low-fat diet for nine unbroken years.

This is not a blanket endorsement that everyone facing a coronary by-pass operation should head for the nearest cardiac rehabilitation center. However, thousands of men and women who had been told by their cardiologists that only surgery could save their lives have gone instead to medically-operated rehabilitation centers and have recovered without surgery or drugs.

Through exercise, they have stimulated the build-up of collateral blood vessels that have by-passed and taken over the function of the blocked arteries. In effect, they have given themselves a by-pass operation without the cost, risk or trauma of surgery.

New Directions in Life Extension

Aging is the result of many factors working at every level in the body and mind. Hence, life can be extended only by a holistic approach using many health-building habits that work on every level to benefit both the mind and body.

These are the primary keys to the holistic approach to health and longevity.

• **We must accept responsibility for our own health and sickness and we must take an active role in reversing disease and in maintaining health.** While this philosophy applies principally to drugs and surgery it also requires us to examine the benefits of non-medical treatments like chiropractic, massage, naturopathy, homeopathy, Rolfing and bodywork, acupuncture, hypnosis and orthomolecular therapy.

The real benefits of holistic healing lie in therapies such as diet, exercise, fasting, meditation, guided imagery, biofeedback, yoga and deep relaxation which we can carry out entirely on our own and without cost.

• **Although licensed holistic practitioners exist, including M.D.s who can be extremely helpful to beginners, holistic healing is essentially a do-it-yourself process based on self-care.** As a result, it costs little or nothing to practice. But to take responsibility for, and to exercise complete control over your own health does require knowledge. Most health seekers are confused by the hundreds of books and magazine articles that offer conflicting holistic philosophies.

Fortunately, the Lifex Constants described in detail in this book also form the basis of the holistic approach to health. Through this book, you will acquire a complete understanding and guide to the holistic approach to health and longevity.

• **All healing is done from within.** Outside practitioners, drugs and surgery cannot heal. They can only treat symptoms. We can heal ourselves only when the causes of illness—our health-destroying habits—are removed. This occurs when through the Lifex Constants, the mind and body are supplied with biological needs such as pure air and water, sound nutrition, exercise, rest, relaxation, security and emotional calm.

• **Failure of the pathology-management industrial complex to produce a cure for any degenerative disease has led to avoidance of the words "health" and "cure" in holistic circles.** "Health," for example, is used interchangably with "disease." Health insurance pays only if you fall sick and most Departments of Health are actually concerned with pathology management.

The average physician is likely to pronounce you in "good health" if a battery of diagnostic tests indicates no signs of illness. "Good health" to most doctors implies not being sick.

To avoid such misuse and misrepresentation, the holistic movement prefers to talk about "wellness." Wellness is not merely an absence of disease. It is a vital state which supplies us with all the energy, vigor, aliveness, and emotional poise we need. It implies having your Whole Person functioning smoothly. It means leading a life designed not merely to produce health but to produce high-level health. To follow a Wellness Lifestyle means that we actively adopt every possible Lifex Constant, not merely the barest minimum.

It is important to remember that the Wellness Lifestyle will provide us with high-level wellness only for as long as we continue to maintain it. Many people, including some physicians, view the Wellness Lifestyle as some form of temporary therapy. After one's weight returns to normal or one's symptoms disappear, they believe that the Wellness Lifestyle can be dropped and we can return to our self-destructive habits.

Such thinking is misleading. The Wellness Lifestyle is a program for life. Dean Ormish, M.D., of Harvard Medical School, found that he could reduce risk of heart disease and incidence of angina in his patients by 90 percent through stress management coupled with a low-fat diet. But after returning to the old habits, or even a single high-fat meal, symptoms returned. Patients who assumed they were "cured," and who stopped the diet and stress management program, found that their chest pains returned. Yet regression was permanent for those who stayed with the program.

The failure of the pathology management industry to achieve a genuine cure for any degenerative disease has caused the holistic movement to talk about "reversal" rather than "cure." As long as we stop abusing ourselves with destructive habits, we are likely to experience a reversal of most degenerative diseases (cancer and other irreversible conditions excepted).

• **Through the holistic approach, you take back your right to control your own life and health.** You do not surrender it to a doctor. In any relationship with a doctor or healer, your role is that of an equal partner, not a dependent while the doctor remains an authority figure. In *High Level Wellness*, author Donald Ardell, Ph.D., writes: "In my opinion (and that of many others), the greatest single cause of poor health in this country is that most Americans neglect, and surrender to others, responsibility for their own health."

A guest editorial in the *American Medical News* stated: "Physicians must recognize that medicine is not their private practice but a profession in which we all have a vital stake." Whereas many centenarians have relied on traditional folk medicine in the past, today we can exert unprecedented control over our own health. Researchers have developed scientifically validated information about how we can reprogram our personality and lifestyle for optimal wellness. Hence, a growing self-care revolution is taking place. Even the government is supporting this trend as evidenced by these words from the Surgeon General in his 1979 report *Health Promotion and Disease Prevention*, "You, the individual, can do more for your own health and well-being than any doctor, any hospital, any drugs, any exotic medical devices."

POSITIVE ACTION STEPS FOR MINIMIZING DEPENDENCE
ON MEDICAL CARE

• Depend on the Wellness Lifestyle to safeguard your health.

• Do not permit reliance on health insurance to influence your incentive to follow the Wellness Lifestyle.

• Avoid all over-the-counter medications. Before asking for tranquilizers, consider such alternatives as exercise, deep relaxation and deep breathing.

• Before agreeing to any but emergency or lifesaving medical care, find out what risks or side effects are involved in the drug or procedure. (Side effects of all prescription drugs are described in the *Physician's Desk Reference*, available in most public libraries.) Find out what alternative, non-medical treatments are available—especially things you could do for yourself. Then ask yourself if you could do without the medical treatment. What would happen if you did not have it?

• Before undergoing any surgery, get a second opinion, preferably from a physician or specialist who is not a surgeon. Consider getting a third opinion from a holistically oriented M.D., or other licensed healing practitioner. Never ask your first doctor to recommend another for a second opinion. Find one who will review your case objectively. You can get free government advice on a second opinion by dialing Second Surgical Opinion Hotline 800-838-6833 (in Maryland 800-492-6603). Many states also have a SSOP (Second Surgical Opinion Program) available to anyone to help verify need for surgery. Write for the booklet *Thinking of Having Surgery*, free from Surgery, Department of Health and Human Services, 200 Independence Avenue S.W., Washington DC 20201.

Because there is often a choice of medical regimens for treating any specific ailment, the average physician may be familiar with only one or two. A second physician may opt to treat you by a less harmful, less expensive and more effective regimen.

• If you *must* undergo surgery or treatment, opt for the minimum possible. If you must take medication, opt for the minimum effective dosage for the shortest possible time.

• If you are already taking medication or undergoing medical procedures, discuss with your doctor the possibility of gradually reducing the dosage as you replace it with such natural therapies as exercise, diet and stress management. If your physician is not receptive to a holistic approach, consider changing to a doctor who is.

• Patronize doctors who are fit and lean, who exercise regularly and who follow a wellness lifestyle themselves. Avoid doctors who are unfamiliar with, or opposed to, the holistic approach to healing. Holistically oriented physicians can now be found in many college towns and in many affluent, less conservative communities where traditional medicine is becoming increasingly suspect.

• If you are on maintenance drugs, or maintenance medical treatment, you should reduce it only under medical supervision. Again, if you are overweight or have any type of dysfunction, obtain your doctor's permission before commencing to exercise, changing your diet or undertaking any other form of natural therapy.

In conjunction with the Lifex Constants in this book, these simple action steps will minimize your dependence on the medical profession. They will boost your incentive to rely on the Wellness Lifestyle. They can save you thousands of dollars in medical bills, and they can add years to your life expectancy.

LIFEX CONSTANT 2: Refrain from Smoking and Using Other Harmful Stimulants

Alcohol, caffeine, nicotine and marijuana are powerful drugs to which we can become painfully addicted. A study at Duke University of 270 older men showed that cigarette smoking was one of the strongest predictors of early death. Smoking pipes, cigars or marijuana can be hazardous; a clear connection has also been established between chewing tobacco and oral cancer.

Tobacco smoke contains acetaldehyde, a potent carcinogen that initiates cancer in the lungs, larynx, esophagus, bladder, kidneys, breast and pancreas. In 1982, U.S. Surgeon General A. Everett Scoop attributed 30 percent of all cancers to smoking. Smokers have a mortality rate double that of non-smokers and they have three times the risk of heart disease. Smoking etches deep lines and wrinkles on the face. It causes rapid aging, osteoporosis, dowager's hump, emphysema and angina spasm, and it lowers HDL levels.

The effects of smoking kill one thousand Americans every day. Almost every smoker eventually contracts emphysema, heart disease or cancer. One British study found that each cigarette smoked shortens life by five and a half minutes and that smoking two packs a day reduces life expectancy by eight years.

The risks of smoking also extend to non-smokers who occupy the same office or household as a smoker. The non-smoking spouse of a heavy smoker faces a loss of four to six years of life expectancy.

Regular, steady drinking also reduces life expectancy by eight years and is associated with a mortality rate two or three times that of non-drinkers. Steady alcohol consumption has been directly linked with cancer of the breast, thyroid, mouth, larynx and esophagus and with cirrhosis of the liver, ulcers, gastritis and suppression of the immune system. It impairs the memory, weakens the heart muscle, and creates digestive disorders. While some studies have shown that moderate drinking elevates HDL levels, a clear causal relationship between moderate alcohol use and long life has not been established. (Moderate drinking is defined as four ounces of 80-proof whiskey, or forty ounces of 4.5 percent beer, or fourteen ounces of wine per day.)

Tea, coffee, chocolate or cola drinks all contain caffeine, a substance high on the list of suspected carcinogens. Coffee doubles risk of heart disease and intensifies angina pain and high blood pressure. People who drink nine or more cups of coffee daily frequently experience chronic tension, anxiety and depression. Caffeine has been implicated as causing benign growths in women's breasts and it lays the groundwork for peptic ulcers and bladder and urinary tract cancer.

Smoking and Alcohol—A Deadly Combination

When two or more stimulants are used together, they form a combination that heightens risk. People who both smoke and drink alcohol have an exceptionally high cancer rate. Cigarette smoking heightens all the risks of caffeine drinking.

The evidence is clear and unmistakable. Stimulants of all kinds are devastating to health. While a single alcoholic drink, or perhaps a single cup of tea per day, might be tolerated, any consumption in excess of these amounts should be regarded as detrimental to health and long life. If you must use alcohol, the safest way is to take a glass of white wine with a meal.

All Stimulants Create Hypoglycemia

Admittedly, steady alcohol indulgence is a disease that requires professional help; however, smoking, caffeine consumption or a mild addiction to alcohol are all habits which can be overcome without difficulty or pain. Some people began indulging in stimulants through peer pressure. Stimulants give a lift that seems to help people cope with stress.

Stimulants create a "high" by causing a rapid rise in blood sugar level. Their effect is identical to that of eating refined carbohydrates like sugar or white flour. Indeed, alcohol *is* a refined carbohydrate and cola drinks are reinforced with sugar to cause blood sugar levels to soar. Smoking and caffeine raise blood sugar levels by triggering release of glycogen (a sugar) from the liver.

In every case, the effect is short-lived. After an hour or so, the blood sugar level comes crashing down and we experience hypoglycemia—low blood sugar level. At this point, we crave more and this elevates our blood sugar level once again.

Among sugars that will raise our blood sugar level rapidly without too many deleterious effects is the fructose in fruit juice. By sipping fruit juice (or by munching a few dried fruits) whenever we feel the need, we can restore our blood sugar level without resorting to harmful foods or stimulants. We can also stabilize the blood sugar level, and prevent hypoglycemia from occurring, by eating a diet composed exclusively of complex carbohydrate foods and low fat protein. (For an explanation of nutritional terms, see Chapter 7.)

Using this information, we can readily overcome all indulgence in stimulants. The basic step is to eliminate all refined carbohydrates and fats from the diet and to replace them with complex carbohydrate foods as described in Lifex Constant 3. Heavy meals should also be avoided while cutting out stimulants (see Lifex Constant 4).

How to End Caffeine and Alcohol Addiction

The caffeine habit is a relatively mild addiction which can be easily overcome. Each day, replace one cup of coffee with a cup of tea. Tea contains approximately half the caffeine content of coffee. Once you have replaced all coffee drinking with tea, begin to replace one cup of tea each day with a cup of herb tea such as linden, peppermint or yerba buena. You may also use fruit juice, carob or carbonated water.

However, sodas or cola drinks should never be used. Fruit juice should be freshly squeezed, or use unsweetened concentrate. Vegetable juices may be substituted if preferred.

Mild alcohol addiction, such as drinking three or four beers each evening, can be overcome by taking one drink less each night until alcohol consumption has been phased out altogether. The alcohol can be replaced with fruit juice or herb teas.

How to Quit Smoking

In *Quit Smoking* by Curtis Casewit (Para Research, 1983), every successful technique for ending tobacco addiction is presented. Thus you may select the method that appeals to you most.

A popular technique is one called the Five Minute Method. It is based on increasing the interval between each cigarette that you smoke by five minutes. You begin with an interval of one hour. The next interval is one hour and five minutes; then one hour and ten minutes; and so on. You also agree not to smoke before breakfast, after dinner, or for one hour after any meal.

Two days before you begin, switch to smoking the brand of cigarettes (or pipe tobacco, cigars, etc.) that you dislike the most. Keep on smoking these until you quit. Have on hand plenty of fruit juice, dried fruits, chewing gum, fresh fruit or anything else you enjoy provided it does not contain sugar, sweetener, caffeine, alcohol or white flour. Finally, make a list of all the reasons why you wish to stop smoking.

Once you begin, the Five Minute Method will cause your smoking to steadily taper off. Assuming you have breakfast at eight, lunch at twelve and dinner at six—and that each meal takes twenty minutes to finish—on the first day you would smoke at 9:20, 10:25, 11:35, 1:20, 2:35, 3:55 and 5:20—a total of seven cigarettes. As the interval between each cigarette steadily widens, you will find yourself gradually tapering off free of any painful withdrawal symptoms.

By the fifth day, you will be smoking only four or five cigarettes. At that point, you will find you can easily quit entirely.

Each morning, as soon as you wake up, read the list of reasons why you wish to quit smoking. Read them also at the end of each meal.

Whenever you feel the need for a cigarette, first take twelve slow, deep breaths. Next, read the list of reasons why you wish to quit. Then sip a glass of fruit juice, chew some gum, or enjoy any of the other harmless cigarette substitutes.

Ten days after beginning the program, you will have completely broken all physical dependence on nicotine. Through Lifex Constants 11, 12 and 13 you can also avoid psychological dependence on smoking. Do not worry if you overeat or put on excess weight. You can work on that later (see Lifex Constant 8). Smoking is such a life-threatening habit that anything else is insignificant in comparison.

Whichever addictions you wish to break, do not postpone starting. Begin as soon as possible and resolve that you are going to overcome the harmful habit. If you fail at first and give in, start right in again immediately.

Rather than view yourself as giving up smoking, caffeine or alcohol, see yourself beginning an exciting, new life as a non-smoker or non-drinker. Within a few days after quitting, your body will begin to detoxify and renew itself. Your sense of smell and taste will return and all your original energy and aliveness will reappear.

Risk of heart disease and emphysema begins to decline immediately when you cease to indulge in stimulants. As the months go by, risk of cancer or other degenerative disease gradually decreases almost to the level of a total abstainer.

7

The Nutritional Approach to Life Extension

Although some centenarians may not consider diet as a principal source of their longevity, an analysis of what they actually eat reveals that many are often vegetarians.

In 1978, on the occasion of her 113 birthday, Mrs. Cynthia Fitzpatrick of Rochester, New York, attributed her long life to a series of Lifex Constants among which a lean diet was paramount. Throughout her life, she had lived almost exclusively on vegetables, fruits and whole grains and had eaten very little meat.

Another healthy, long-lived American, Wally Latimer, who was still operating a Kansas farm when he turned 98 a few years ago, said that living almost entirely on fruits and vegetables had helped him to remain at 130 pounds throughout his active life.

The world's longest-lived man, Shigechiyo Izumi of Japan, who died in 1981, had eaten vegetables, cereals and beans, supplemented by small amounts of fresh fish, for most of his 116 years.

LIFEX CONSTANT 3: Follow Sound Nutritional Practices

A low consumption of animal protein, fat and refined carbohydrates is a Lifex Constant found in almost all studies of healthy, long-lived people. Vegetarian groups such as the Vegans, Natural Hygienists, Seventh Day Adventists and followers of a macrobiotic diet all show levels of blood pressure, heart disease, cancer and diabetes far below the average in the United States. These findings are also supported by numerous studies which indicate that diets which are predominently or exclusively vegetarian lead to an increase of several years in life expectancy.

It was the Worldwatch Organization of Washington D.C., that first drew attention to the hazards of the standard American diet by linking the leading causes of non-accidental death in the United States with the fat, meat, dairy products and processed foods we eat. A series of subsequent reports then followed, each increasingly pointing to our consumption of animal-derived foods and refined flour and sugar as being the major cause of heart disease, cancer, diabetes and other diseases.

The National Institutes of Health set the pace by endorsing *The Alternative Diet Book*, which recommended drastic reductions in meat and a corresponding increase in consumption of vegetable dishes.

In 1977, the Senate Committee on Nutrition and Human Needs published *Eating in America: Dietary Goals For the U.S.*, which urged Americans to cut consumption of fat, meat, dairy foods, eggs and sugar by 40 percent and to replace them with increasing amounts of fresh fruits and vegetables.

The message was repeated in 1979 in *Healthy People*, the Surgeon General's report on health promotion, which associated consumption of animal protein and fat with incidence of atherosclerosis, heart disease and several types of cancer. Americans were advised to cut down on fat, sugar and salt, to replace meat with vegetables and beans, and to consume only sufficient calories to meet the body's needs.

In 1982, the National Academy of Sciences released their *Diet, Nutrition and Cancer* report, which announced that Americans could reduce risk of breast and colon cancer by reducing their daily fat intake and by avoiding foods cured by smoking, salting or pickling. The gist of the report was that a low-fat, high-fiber diet of fresh fruits, vegetables, seeds, beans and whole grains—especially green and yellow vegetables—has been shown to deter several common forms of cancer.

In the same year, the Ford Foundation commissioned renowned nutritionist Joseph Beasley, M.D., to set nutritional guidelines for its health and education programs. Dr. Beasley's report, entitled *The Impact of Nutrition on the Health of Americans* stated that the nation's health is being destroyed by our high consumption of fat, sugar and processed foods.

Gremlin Foods That Destroy Our Health

The news that pizza, hamburgers, ice cream, and hot dogs can shorten our lives has become an emotionally charged issue. Food is often equated with love when offered as a gift or when served at social events. In fact, the daily lives of Americans often revolve around eating foods that may eventually kill them.

Yet the threat to our health and well-being is so great that Dr. William P. Castelli, director of the Framingham Heart Study, has stated that "the cornerstone to protecting your health is diet. Most problems affecting our aging are the chronic degenerative diseases and we have to recognize that three-fourths of the people on earth don't get these diseases. When we eat a diet that is sparse in meats and fats we do a lot better."

Dr. Castelli also pointed out that "vegetarians are at a much lower risk from heart disease than meat eaters. Study after study has clearly demonstrated the value of a vegetarian diet in combating heart disease."

As Dr. Castelli pointed out, hundreds of important studies have linked certain foods to degenerative diseases. By combining the results of all of these studies, scientists have been able to develop diets that help prevent disease. Other nutritionists like Dr. Arnold Fox and Nathan Pritikin have developed nutritionally sound diets that eliminate obesity and that will maintain a person's weight at the optimal level throughout life.

As details of these various diets become known, scientists began to note a rather curious fact. For example, a group of experimental biologists at the University of California, San Diego, were among the first to note that the same low-fat diet of natural vegetarian foods recommended to prevent all forms of cardiovascular disease was virtually identical with the diet recommended to prevent cancer. These diets were essentially the same as all the other diets that had been scientifically demonstrated to eliminate diabetes, glaucoma, diverticulosis, gallstones, kidney stones and obesity.

One Diet Does It All

Gerontologists noticed that this diet was the same vegetarian diet of fresh fruits, vegetables, nuts, seeds and whole grains that had been eaten by the majority of healthful centenarians throughout their lives. Nutritional authorities now believe that this diet will lead to optimal wellness and enhanced longevity.

The evidence is clear and unmistakable. Our bodies are not adapted to many of the foods we eat. Our digestive system was inherited from primate ancestors who lived on fruits, vegetables, nuts, seeds, roots and grains. When we punish our bodies by feeding them meat, fat and refined flour and sugar, our cells rebel. Eventually, our arteries become clogged with cholesterol and we may experience a stroke or heart attack; or our cells become engorged with fat and we get diabetes; or our cells become mutant and we are prone to cancer.

Amazingly, however, the body can recuperate from much of the damage caused by these foods in just a short time. Surveys have shown that meat eaters who switch to a vegetarian diet can significantly reduce risk of heart attack in weeks. Cholesterol levels drop dramatically as soon as we cease to eat saturated fats. Many cases of Type II diabetes have been controlled when patients changed to vegetarian diets.

Revolution in Nutrition

Vegetarianism is not a diet. It is a philosophy for healthful eating that eliminates all foods of animal origin plus all refined and processed foods. There remains a wide choice of delicious foods from which to choose at every meal.

To make the transition into vegetarianism smoother, a modified vegetarian diet will allow you to continue to eat some of the least harmful foods of animal origin such as fish, egg whites and low-fat dairy foods. Some people never get beyond this modified vegetarian diet. They are content to stay with it and in the process they reduce their intake of harmful foods well below the levels recommended by government studies.

Yet, if you are a dedicated health seeker, intent on attaining exceptional health and maximum longevity, you will eventually want to adopt a totally vegetarian diet.

Vegetarianism implies more than merely eliminating foods of animal origin. It includes eliminating all foods that are harmful to the human body, particularly foods that are processed, refined, preserved, manufactured, canned, fragmented, smoked, salted or pickled. It includes eating as many foods as possible in a fresh and uncooked state. It includes minimizing cooking and it implies total elimination of all fried foods, fast foods and convenience foods. It includes learning to enjoy the taste of natural foods without disguising them with commercial mayonnaise, sauces, ketchup, salt, pepper or other condiments. It includes learning how to maximize the enjoyment of eating without overeating or eating compulsively. It includes the ability to distinguish between natural foods that benefit the Whole Person and non-foods such as sugar, white flour and fat.

This healthful form of vegetarianism excludes the lacto-ovo variety of vegetarianism (which allows eggs and dairy products). It views the macrobiotic vegetarian diet (based largely on grains) as being deficient in vegetables and fruit. True vegetarianism is based on eating a balanced diet consisting of twice as many vegetables as fruits plus some whole grains, nuts and seeds. Grains and legumes may be cooked but, ideally, they are better sprouted. It is this form of vegetarianism, which eliminates all pressed vegetable oils and fats, that the Framingham Heart Study found to provide great protection against heart disease.

Counterfeit Foods

Most newcomers to nutrition are so confused by contrary reports regarding various foods that they find it extremely difficult to make informed choices. Since the FTC recently killed a nine-year-old proposal to require disclosure of specific content information for foods advertised as low in cholesterol, calories or fat, food manufacturers have launched gigantic advertising campaigns to promote high-fat foods as healthful, highly processed foods as natural, and high-calorie foods as weight reducing.

Overlaying such deception are extravagent claims for various "wonder foods" supposed to restore youth and health and to extend life. Millions of people are misled daily, for example, when they buy commercial "whole wheat" bread with the belief that it is good for their health. In actuality, most "whole wheat" bread sold in supermarkets is made *with* whole wheat flour, not *exclusively of* whole wheat flour, and the loaf typically contains such high-risk foods as white flour, sugar, fat, oils, eggs and chemical additives.

Nor is orthodox nutrition, with its dependence on eating from the four basic food groups, entirely dependable. A study made in 1981 at Pennsylvania State University (reported in the *Journal of Nutrition Education*, Vol 13, #2, 1981) found that the food choices of 212 young adults for one day—including 46 who ate the recommended number of servings from all four food groups—showed that 66 percent of the 212 had an intake below the RDA (recommended daily allowance) for Vitamins E and B_6, iron and zinc. One-third also tested low in folate and magnesium. Similar tests have shown that when given free choice between wholesome foods and sweets, both children and adults, and also animals, usually choose sweets.

To learn to eat successfully we must first become familiar with the pros and cons of the three types of food—carbohydrates, fat and protein.

CARBOHYDRATES

Carbohydrates supply the body with energy, primarily in the form of sugar or starch. All foods of vegetable origin including fruits, vegetables, nuts, seeds, legumes, tubers and grains consist predominently of carbohydrates. It is, therefore, important to distinguish between complex, unrefined carbohydrates and simple, refined carbohydrates.

Complex (Unrefined) Carbohydrates refer to any vegetable food in its whole, original, unrefined and unprocessed state in which the cells are enclosed in a membrane of cellulose. Complex carbohydrates are also known as *living foods* because their cells are still alive. The cells of all fruits, vegetables, nuts, seeds, beans, tubers and grains remain alive for as long as the food is fit to eat. Many of these foods when planted in the ground will begin to grow. Some grains, such as oatmeal, are sliced. Whole wheat, for example, may be ground into flour. Such mildly processed whole grain products retain their cellulose content and also retain the qualities of living foods before they begin to spoil.

Since cellulose cannot be digested by humans, all forms of complex carbohydrates break down at a slow, steady pace in the stomach and intestines.

Their nutrients are thus absorbed at a gradual rate that keeps the blood sugar level constantly stabilized.

Simple (Refined) Carbohydrates are created when the cells of sugar, grain or rice are stripped of their cellulose walls to increase their shelf life. When wheat is refined into white flour, the entire germ of the wheat is destroyed along with almost all fiber, Vitamin B$_6$, magnesium and manganese. Refined flour and sugar constitute empty calories. Bakers attempt to restore some of the nutrients by enriching white bread with synthetic vitamins, but they cannot restore the fiber.

Unlike complex carbohydrates whose fiber (cellulose) content retards absorption, white flour and sugar (sucrose) are absorbed rapidly by the intestines, sending blood sugar and insulin levels soaring and elevating both triglycerides and cholesterol levels. Several studies have proved that repeated consumption of refined carbohydrates makes the body more vulnerable to diabetes and heart disease and to increased damage from smoking, alcohol, drugs and radiation.

A 1983 study by dietician Phyllis Crapo of Stanford University showed that, when eaten alone, some types of refined carbohydrates were absorbed more slowly, and raised blood sugar levels less, than some types of complex carbohydrates. However, like most research which tests only a single variable, the study failed to consider the effects of the fiber, nutrient and calorie content of various cabohydrate foods. The study ignored the effect of carbohydrates in the context of a full meal, which also includes fats and protein. For example, digestion of any carbohydrate can be slowed by adding fat. The form of carbohydrates, the extent of processing, and the degree of exposure to heat during cooking, also affect the rate at which carbohydrates are absorbed and the rate at which they increase blood sugar and insulin levels. Again, the study considered only short-term results and overlooked the harmful results of eating refined carbohydrates over a longer period. Most major nutritional advisory groups have cautioned Americans to beware of recommendations based on these studies, which may suggest that we can now safely eat more fats and refined carbohydrates without increasing risk of heart disease, diabetes or other degenerative diseases.

We should also be aware that all forms of sweeteners are refined carbohydrates including honey, brown sugar, beet sugar, molasses, all syrups, dextrin, galactose, lactose, malt, sorbitol, sorghum, xylose and extracted fructose. Dried fruits are also refined carbohydrates and should be eaten sparingly. By dramatically elevating blood sugar and insulin levels, eating refined carbohydrates may lead to hypoglycemia and sugar addiction.

Widespread craving for sugar and white flour has led manufacturers to include them in almost all types of canned, processed, manufactured and prepared foods. Even baby foods often contain these undesirable ingredients.

In eating for long life, all refined carbohydrates should be avoided, and complex carbohydrates in the form of fresh, raw and whole (uncut) fruits, vegetables, seeds, nuts and whole grains should be included in our diet. Whole grain flours, and especially oatmeal, are acceptable but always choose those which are most coarsely cut or ground.

Buttress Your Diet with Fiber

Numerous studies have shown that dietary fiber, found only in complex carbohydrates, is healthful. In 1982, the National Academy of Sciences recommended a high intake of dietary fiber at all three meals as a cancer preventative. All diets recommended to prevent or reverse degenerative diseases are high in fiber because fiber has been shown to prevent absorption of fat and cholesterol.

Fiber does not exist in foods of animal origin and in refined carbohydrates. Cooking destroys fiber in all foods but grains. Hence we must look for fiber in living foods, especially in such whole grains as brown rice, kasha, bulgur wheat and steamed millet. Fiber may also be found in green, leafy vegetables; in cabbage-family vegetables like Brussels sprouts, brocoli and cauliflower; and in carrots, legumes, tubers and hard fruits like apples. A breakfast dish of oatmeal sprinkled with slices of unpeeled apples provides a combination that sweeps fat and cholesterol through the intestines.

Adding bran to the standard American diet will help to prevent constipation. But adding bran will not lower levels of fat and cholesterol in the bloodstream. Only a diet of complex carbohydrates can do that. Granola is not recommended due to its high content of oils and sweeteners. Most commercial breakfast cereals, of course, are simply candy in disguise. Among the few wholesome cereals sold on supermarket shelves are Nabisco's Shredded Wheat, Kellogg's Nutri-grain series and the Swiss Muesli.

The cellulose, lignum, gum and pectin that comprise fiber sweep through the intestines and are eliminated in a mere twenty-four to thirty hours. In comparison, it takes 3 or 4 days for a low residue diet of animal products, refined carbohydrates and highly cooked foods to accomplish this. Dietary fiber expands stool volume between two and four and a half times, making stools large, soft, and easily passed. Most vegetarians do not experience constipation.

Because dietary fiber soaks up fat and cholesterol and inhibits their absorption by the body, a complex carbohydrate diet prevents weight gain.

You can eat all the complex carbohydrates you want, including starches, and restore your weight to normal.

FATS

Fat refers to the fatty acids derived from foods that help support and insulate the body, that transport the fat-soluble Vitamins A, D and E and that, when broken down into lipids in the body, perform several important biochemical functions. Four basic types of fat are found in foods: saturated, polyunsaturated, mono-unsaturated and hydrogenated fats.

Saturated Fats have a carbon skeleton that is saturated by carrying its maximum capacity of hydrogen atoms. All saturated fats are of animal origin and have a melting point between 100°-109°F. This means that cholesterol, found only in saturated fats, remains solid when deposited in the arteries and causes atherosclerosis and cardiovascular disease. Because cattle in the United States are bred to produce marbled meats throughout the body, the standard American diet is dangerously high in saturated fats. The United States still has one of the world's highest rates of cardiovascular disease.

Polyunsaturated Fats have a carbon skeleton consisting of double bonds in which one or more spots remain unfilled by hydrogen atoms. All polyunsaturated fats are of vegetable origin and exist in their natural form in avocadoes, legumes, nuts, seeds and grains. However, the largest source of dietary unsaturated fats are oils squeezed from grains, seeds, legumes and olives. All polyunsaturated fats are liquid at body temperature, hence they do not create arterial blocks. But actual melting points range all the way from 98°F for peanut butter to only 49°F for fish body oils.

Recent studies in Denmark, Japan and the United States have revealed that, when eaten, fish body oils reduce the LDL (low density lipoprotein) level, cause a large reduction in cholesterol and triglycerides, inhibit platelet clumping and relieve angina pains. Fish body oils are obtained by eating fish and seafood. Fish-eating peoples, including Eskimo, Japanese fishermen, Icelanders and Norwegians, all have a low incidence of cardiovascular disease.

However, the principal hazard of polyunsaturated fat is that it oxidizes rapidly when exposed to air and becomes chemically rancid, a condition that occurs without affecting its taste. Hence its rancidity passes unnoticed. Once a polyunsaturated fat becomes rancid, free radicals are released that transform the oil into a cancer activator inside the body.

Thus, while marine oils from the bodies of fish and crustacae may prevent cardiovascular disease, their presence in the human body could increase risk of cancer or diabetes. Fish is a high-protein food and protein from animal sources has been linked with increased risk of both cancer and heart disease.

Nonetheless, of all animal foods, fish, shellfish, lobster and shrimp etc., (but not roe or fish organs) appear among the least harmful.

Polyunsaturated oils are frequently used in frying, cooking and baking and are a key ingredient in hundreds of common processed and prepared foods.

Mono-Unsaturated Fat, principally olive oil, has a melting point of 82 °F but its molecular structure is such that it contains only 10 to 15 percent as much linoleic acid as most polyunsaturated fats. Linoleic acid, the only fatty acid which cannot be synthesized by the body, is now suspected of contributing to cardiovascular disease. People who traditionally consume large amounts of olive oil, such as the Greeks and Italians, have an exceptionally low rate of heart disease. For example, Greek men aged 55 to 65 have one-tenth the heart disease of American men of the same age. Greeks take between 15 and 30 percent of their calories from olive oil, which has a low content of linoleic acid and a high content of oleic acid. Oleic acid is believed to reduce the body's LDL level.

Hydrogenated Fats consist of polyunsaturated oils into which hydrogen atoms have been forced to make them solid. Through modern technology, any degree of hydrogenation may be achieved. Thus, oils may be only partially-hydrogenated. Any degree of hydrogenation causes oil to change its molecular structure and become a trans-fatty acid. Oils are hydrogenated to prevent rancidity and to increase their shelf life. This artificial processing makes hydrogenated fats extremely dangerous to eat.

Hydrogenated, or partially hydrogenated, oils have a higher cholesterol content than natural fats and have been identified as a major risk-factor for atherosclerosis, platelet clumping, heart disease, stroke, and hypertension. They have no nutritional benefit and interfere with the normal activity of the body's enzymes, hormones and prostaglandins. Obviously, these processed fats should never be consumed under any circumstances. Yet processed fats are commonly found in manufactured peanut butter, salad dressing, vegetable shortening, margarine and commercial breads and baked goods. You can often identify foods that contain hydrogenated vegetable oils because they are also frequently loaded with sugar and salt.

The Health Hazards of a High-Fat Diet

Early in the 1950s, scientists discovered that cholesterol in saturated fats was the prime cause of arterial blockage and most forms of cardiovascular disease. Americans were advised to replace saturated fats in the diet with polyunsaturated fats. The result was a steady decline in cardiovascular disease and a corresponding rise in the incidence of cancer. Until the early 1980s, scientists were unaware that polyunsaturated fat could be the major activator of cancer.

Meanwhile, all fats are suspected of contributing to other degenerative diseases. Throughout the world, the higher the fat intake, the higher the rate of heart disease, diabetes and all forms of cancer.

Thus, it is not merely saturated fats that must be reduced in the diet. All forms of fat are considered hazardous to health. Even fish oils and olive oil—while beneficial to the cardiovascular system—may well be cancer activators and could contribute to diabetes and other chronic diseases.

The body actually needs very little fat. With the exception of linoleic acid, we can synthesize all other fatty acids we require from complex carbohydrates. Our daily requirement of linoleic acid can easily be met by a small bowl of oatmeal.

In experiments which reduced symptoms of heart disease and angina by 90 percent, Dean Ormish, M.D., of Harvard Medical School, cut cholesterol intake in his patients to a mere 5 mgs daily. The American average is between 450 and 600 mgs. Similar results have been obtained by Nathan Pritikin and by other cardiologists in charge of cardiac rehabilitation centers. When fat was cut from 40 percent of calorie intake (as in the standard American diet), to only 10 percent or less, patients experienced dramatic improvements in as little as two or three weeks.

Numerous studies have shown that most people have no physiological need for the high levels of fat in the standard American diet. The Food and Nutrition Board of the National Academy of Sciences has recommended a minimum fat intake of only 1 or 2 percent of total calories (equivalent to one teaspoon of oil or butter per day). This is all the fat we need to remain healthy. Several other studies have found that whenever more than 15 percent of a person's daily calories are derived from fat, facial wrinkles begin to appear, fatigue increases, atherosclerosis manifests, and fat begins to interfere with the efficiency of the immune system.

All this has led progressive nutritionists to recommend that we limit our fat intake to only 5 or 10 percent of our daily calories. In practice, our need for fat can be safely met by our normal consumption of grains, seeds, nuts, legumes and avocadoes. We have no need for vegetable oils, animal fats, dairy foods or fried foods of any type. Even fish, seafood and olive oil should be eaten sparingly.

PROTEIN

Protein consists of twenty-two different amino acids, which form the building blocks of the body. Of these, our bodies can synthesize fourteen amino acids from other foods. The remaining eight, known as *essential amino acids*, must be obtained from food. Complete protein is obtainable from both animal and vegetarian sources. All animal protein contains the eight essential amino acids and is considered to be whole protein. No single vegetarian food contains all eight. But foods such as nuts, seeds, legumes and grains each contain different essential amino acids. Our daily protein requirements are easily met by a well-complemented mix of seeds, peas, beans, nuts and whole grains plus sprouts of any kind.

According to United Nation's nutritional studies, an adult requires only .37 grams of animal protein or .51 grams of plant protein per pound of body weight per day. This works out to a daily need for approximately two and a half ounces of plant protein by a 130-pound woman and three ounces by a 160-pound man. Vegetarians easily meet these requirements by including in their diets an assortment of such foods as brown rice, corn, oatmeal, beans, seeds and sprouts. Essential amino acids lacking in one food are supplied by another. Methionine, for example, which is low in legumes, is plentifully supplied by whole grains.

The standard American diet supplies approximately three times as much protein as we actually need. Cancers of the lymph system, brain and nervous system, as well as progressive bone loss, have all been associated with excessive intake of animal protein. Animal protein promotes rapid growth, and large body size increases cancer risk. Meat and other growth-producing foods such as dairy products, eggs, seafood, fish and poultry have been linked to at least half of all male cancers and to over two-thirds of female cancers.

The Danger of Excessive Protein

Other researchers such as Dr. K.K. Carroll of the University of Western Ontario have found a relationship between animal protein and heart disease that corresponds exactly to the relationship found between cholesterol and heart disease. Animal protein is usually associated with fat, but even animal protein that has been totally separated from fat has increased serum cholesterol levels.

The same effect is apparent in milk and dairy products. Skim milk and low-fat yogurt or cottage cheese provide a relatively fat-free source of whole protein. But even without their fat content, milk and dairy products may be harmful. A 1979 study at the University of California, Berkeley, found that the amino acid tryptophan, which exists in milk and dairy products, sends signals to the pituitary gland that are believed to accelerate physical aging throughout the body.

Several more recent studies have found that milk and dairy products contain estradiol, a hormone that promotes rapid growth in calves. In a study of fifteen hundred women with benign breast lumps at the University of British Columbia, Dr. L.B. Franklin reportedly found that estradiol apparently leads to breast disease in women who consume large amounts of cheese or other dairy products. When the women cut out dairy foods altogether, 85 percent became free of breast lumps and the majority also lost significant weight.

Another study of 122 men aged 61 to 88 found that those who had experienced heart attacks had significantly higher levels of estradiol in their bloodstream than those who had not. Of the fifteen with the highest estradiol level, thirteen had had heart attacks.

Today, more and more nutritionists are beginning to concur that milk may be a fine food for calves but should not be consumed by humans.

Study after study is continuing to confirm the risks of eating animal protein. A typical seven-year study of eleven thousand people—43 percent of whom were vegetarian—by the Medical Research Council Epidemiology Unit at Cardiff, Wales, found that the meat-eating men in the study had one and a half times the death rate of those who ate only plant protein. Animal protein has also been identified as decreasing the amount of serotonin in the brain, thereby increasing risk of sudden cardiac death.

Protein from plant sources, by contrast, is high in fiber and inhibits absorption of cholesterol and other fats through the intestines. Thus, plant protein protects us against cardiovascular disease, cancer, diabetes and most forms of degenerative disease.

Extending Life with Living Foods

After reviewing the results of nutritional studies from around the world, the National Academy of Sciences in 1982 recommended that Americans eat a diet high in living foods. Each day we should eat at least three ounces of foods containing beta-carotene, a precursor of Vitamin A. Beta-carotene is essential for maintenance of epithelium (skin) cells that cover most organ and body passageways and where more than half of all cancers occur. Foods rich in beta-carotene are carrots and carrot juice; dark, green, leafy vegetables; dark yellow and red fruits and vegetables; and yellow-orange fruits like canteloupes, peaches and papaya.

The National Academy also recommended daily consumption of substantial amounts of foods containing indoles, which have been found to prevent formation of breast, stomach and other cancers. Indoles are found in all cabbage family vegetables including Brussels sprouts, cauliflower and broccoli.

Also recommended is daily consumption of seed and tuber vegetables that will grow if planted. A seventeen-year study by Japan's National Research Center found that eating beans, tubers, seeds, and green and yellow vegetables led to significantly lower rates of hypertension, cardiovascular disease, gastric ulcers and many common types of cancer. Walter Troll, professor of Medicine at New York University, reported to the American Cancer Society in 1983, that enzymes in all forms of seeds and tubers have inhibited development of several common forms of cancer. Seeds, he explained, contain protease inhibitors that work with body enzymes to prevent tumor formation. (Every type of vegetable, seed, nut and grain which will grow if planted in the ground is a seed by definition.)

Curiously, all these discoveries lacked funding for further research by United States institutions. However, in countries like Japan and Britain where state-subsidized research is available, studies continue to confirm that people who eat large amounts of vegetables and little or no animal foods have a very low incidence of degenerative diseases. Fruits like apples, pears, grapes and peaches contain pectin, which helps eliminate cholesterol deposits. Most living foods, especially the white rinds of citrus fruits, contain bioflavinoids, which help restore youthful elasticity to aging arteries.

Eating the 80-10-10 Way

Based on these nutritional discoveries, we can begin to eat for longer life by applying the 80-10-10 formula developed by Nathan Pritikin, founder of the Longevity Research Institute at Santa Monica, California. The center eliminates all fats, oils, fatty meats, refined carbohydrates, sweeteners, salt and caffeine. It limits foods derived from animals to negligible amounts while boosting intake of complex carbohydrates rich in fiber and nutrients.

The 80-10-10 formula implies that 80 percent of your daily calorie intake should consist of complex carbohydrates (fresh fruits, vegetables, sprouts, whole grains); not more than 10 percent should consist of fat (ideally from seeds, nuts and avocadoes); and only 10 percent should come from protein (preferably from plant sources; otherwise from low fat dairy products, fish, or poultry minus the skin).

Many people who eat for health and long life plan their menus so that breakfast is primarily a fruit meal, lunch is primarily protein, and dinner primarily starch. A typical menu might be oatmeal and fresh fruit for breakfast; a bean-rice-cereal combination followed by sunflower and sesame seeds with a grapefruit for lunch; and a large vegetable salad followed by a dish of lightly steamed starchy vegetables like sweet potatoes, squash, beets and rutabagas for dinner. Baked potatoes could be added. Natural seasonings such as garlic, lemon juice, herbs and onions are used in place of salt, condiments and commercial sauces and dressings.

Because most hot meals contain meat and people still believe that meat is full of "goodness," the hot meal has become incorrectly associated with wholesome eating. In reality, heat adds nothing to food and merely destroys fiber, enzymes and vitamins. Frying multiplies calories in any food. A potato that contains only 100 calories contains 300 if fried and 500 when converted into potato chips. So steam, broil or bake instead of frying. Do not be afraid to eat living foods containing starch. Starch in complex carbohydrates is not fattening. It is the cream and butter we put on potatoes that make calories soar.

For optimum nutrition, many foods should be eaten raw. People who eat for long life regard a salad as the main course at each meal. Almost all fruits and vegetables plus nuts, seeds and sprouts can be made into delicious salads and eaten raw. Since vegetables contain twice as many nutrients as fruits, try to eat twice as many vegetables as fruits. Mix colors in salads, and when steaming vegetables, so that you have plenty of green, yellow and red vegetables. Darker vegetables contain more minerals and enzymes. Romaine and other loose leaf lettuce is preferable to the tightly packed Iceberg variety which lacks chlorophyll. Use sharp, peppery vegetables like green onions, watercress, mustard and radish in small amounts to add flavor.

Healthful Eating

By following these rules for eating, we can rediscover the honest taste of natural foods. Most Americans are so accustomed to disguising the taste of denatured foods with a variety of sauces, dressings and condiments that they can no longer enjoy the taste of unadulterated food. Every year, those who eat the standard American diet consume a total of at least five pounds of chemical food additives, used in almost all preserved, processed, canned and convenience foods. Almost every canned and packaged food on supermarket shelves contains a host of preservatives, dyes, stabilizers and bleaching, texturizing and taste enhancing agents that mask disagreeable tastes or restore bright colors and crispness to limp, faded foods. Up to six hundred different chemicals are also used in processing meat and poultry.

A 1979 report by the U.S. General Accounting Office found that 14 percent of dressed meat and poultry sold in supermarkets may contain illegally high residues of chemicals suspected to be carcinogenic or capable of producing birth defects. Only a handful of the five thousand chemical additives commonly used have been tested for safety by the FDA. No long-term testing for cancer, birth defects or other toxic risks is ever made nor are the hazards of mixing one additive with another ever considered.

This danger alone should be sufficient to cause us to avoid foods which are not sold in whole, natural, and unprocessed conditions. For health and long life, you should confine your shopping entirely to the produce section of your supermarket, to the bins in your local grainary, or to other whole, natural food stores, which have not tampered with or processed the foods.

Easy Transition into the Healthful Diet

Rather than suddenly giving up all unhealthy foods at once, you can smooth your transition into a living-food diet. The first day, eat one fruit before beginning your regular breakfast, after which you can eat as much of your regular breakfast as you desire. Eat a small vegetable salad before beginning on your regular lunch and dinner. Eat only until you feel satisfied and try to leave some of your regular meal unfinished. The second day, eat two fruits before your regular breakfast and increase the size of the lunch and dinner salads. The third day, eat three fruits at breakfast and keep increasing the lunch and dinner salads. On the fourth day, eat four fruits at breakfast and eat a large salad before the other meals. From then on, you can drop all unhealthy foods and stay with a diet entirely composed of living foods.

If this does not sound feasible, consider a modified living-foods diet. This means that you include as many living foods in your diet as you can, but you supplement them with small amounts of animal-derived and other foods. Among these foods are tofu and similar soy products, just about all fish and seafood, chicken or turkey without the skin, wild game or range-bred cattle, skim milk, kefir, buttermilk, low-fat cottage cheese and plain, low-fat yogurt free of gelatin; egg whites; baker's, farmer's and hoop cheese; pancakes, bread and baked goods made exclusively with whole grain flour and egg whites and free of oils and sweeteners; corn tortillas; and home-made low-fat salad dressings. Animal, fish and poultry organs should never be eaten.

Several cookbooks are available containing vegetarian recipes and other recipes low in fat and animal protein. All these can help decondition you from continuing to eat the standard American diet. After staying with the modified living-foods diet for a few weeks, many health seekers have found it easy to switch to a total diet of living foods.

LIFEX CONSTANT 4: Eat Sparingly

There is growing evidence that excess food overloads the body's metabolism. A variety of important studies have all shown that a diet low in calories, fat and animal protein will prevent, and often reverse, most chronic diseases. A frugal eating system devised by Dr. Roy C. Walford, an aging specialist at UCLA Medical School, is the most significant technique so far developed that retards aging, reduces risk of disease, and may extend life by several years.

Since the sixteenth century when Luigi Cornaro lived to be 97 through eating a spare diet, scientists have suspected that reducing food intake can lengthen life in both animals and humans. Convincing evidence came in 1928 when Clive McCay of Cornell University compared a group of free-feeding rats with another group fed only one-third as many calories but with a full spectrum of vitamins and minerals. The oldest animals in the free-feeding group lived only 969 days compared to an average of 1,465 days for the calorie-restricted group. More recent studies at the Chase Institute for Cancer Research, Memorial Sloan-Kettering Cancer Center, and the University of London have all confirmed that frugal eating extends the life of lab animals by up to 50 percent or more and reduces incidence of all types of chronic disease.

As described in Chapter 2 ("Cholesterol Theory of Aging"), reduced intake of food also limits cholesterol production by the liver. As a result, atherosclerosis and many other common symptoms of aging are postponed while risk of heart disease and stroke are greatly reduced.

Dr. Roy C. Walford, who developed the Immunological Theory of Aging, found that when calorie intake is gradually reduced by one-third (while intake of all thirty-two essential vitamins and minerals is maintained at normal levels), shrinking of the thymus gland is slowed. As a result, the immune system remains younger longer with decreased risk of cancer, infections and auto-immune diseases. Other tests have demonstrated that a lean diet minimizes the number of free radicals in the body and reduces the aging effects of cross-linkage. The metabolic rate of the entire body slows and activity of the neuro-endocrine system declines.

When these studies are extrapolated to humans, most show that the younger the age at which we begin to eat a lean diet, the longer we can expect to live. However, a growing number of lab-animal studies are also showing that even when frugal eating is begun in middle age, normal life expectancy is extended by 10 or 15 percent or more.

These results all confirm a Lifex Constant found in virtually all longe-vous people, namely that they never overeat and they stop eating before they are full.

You can put this powerful life extension technique to work almost immediately by starting a gradual decrease in overall calorie intake.

Reduce Your Calorie Intake

To calculate your actual daily calorie intake needs, multiply your *desirable* body weight by 15 and subtract 10 for every year you are over 35. For a 60-year-old man with a desirable weight of 170 pounds, the calculation would be: $170 \times 15 - 250 = 2,300$ calories (the maximum allowable daily intake). However, if you exercise a great deal, you can increase this multiple from 15 to as high as 20. If you take no exercise at all, you can reduce the multiple to as low as 10. The 2,300 calories in the example compares with the adult American male's average intake of 3,300 calories per day.

(Note: The American Heart Association recommends using the 1959 Metropolitan Life Insurance Company's height-weight table to arrive at your desirable weight instead of the newer and more liberal 1983 table. The 1959 table assumes persons are wearing three and a half pounds of clothing, men are wearing one-inch heels and women two-inch heels. To reduce 1983 weights back to 1959 levels, subtract these amounts from the 1983 chart. *Women:* short, 10 lbs; medium height, 8 lbs; tall, 3 lbs. *Men:* short, 13 lbs; medium height, 7 lbs; tall, 2 lbs.)

Dr. Walford advises that you decrease calorie intake very gradually over a period of three or four years from your present intake level. Obviously, you would make your earliest cuts in fat, refined carbohydrates and other harmful foods. Protein intake should not be cut below 10 percent of daily calorie intake.

While we are gradually reducing calorie intake over the recommended three- or four-year period, we can achieve more rapid benefits by using the following four techniques.

1. **Eat only when actually hungry.** This practice has been successfully followed by many healthy centenarians.

2. **Fast one day per week.** Many long-lived people have made a practice of skipping all meals on one day each week. This technique reduces your weekly calorie intake by 14 percent.

3. **Eat meals which are high in complex carbohydrates.** Due to their fibrous bulk, complex carbohydrates satisfy hunger and satiety mechanisms before any appreciable calorie intake has been consumed.

4. **Divide your three regular meals into five to ten mini meals eaten at regular intervals throughout the day.** Eating large meals speeds arrival and absorption of glucose in the intestines and triggers an immediate craving for still more food. Our primate ancestors nibbled small amounts of food at frequent intervals. Hence, our bodies were never designed to handle the stress of coping with large, heavy meals. Digesting a large meal increases the heart rate by twenty to thirty beats per minute and causes abrupt increases in blood sugar level, insulin secretion and cholesterol production. A two-year study of 4,057 people aged 20 and over by Dr. Allen B. Nicholls at the University of Michigan revealed that eating large meals was as dangerous to the heart as eating a high-fat diet.

But when our three standard meals are divided up into ten smaller meals, the reduced body stress significantly lowers risk of heart disease. This conclusion was arrived at by Dr. Grant Gwineup, a professor at the University of California, Irvine, when he changed meal patterns in a student group from three regular meals to ten mini meals eaten at equally-spaced intervals throughout the day. A similar study by Dr. Paul Fabry of Prague University, Czechoslovakia, found that heart disease was greater among men aged 60 to 64 who ate three or fewer meals a day (30.5 percent had heart attacks) than among those who consumed the same ration spread over five or more meals (only 20 percent had heart attacks). Dr. Fabry found that eating large meals can lead to hypertension, cardiovascular disease, diabetes and suppression of the immune system.

You can easily begin eating the mini-meal way by dividing each of your standard meals into two or three smaller meals. The overall daily calorie consumption remains unchanged, but benefits become apparent quickly. Medically supervised tests have shown, for instance, that overweight people who switch to a mini-meal routine frequently lose two pounds per week without reducing calorie intake. High cholesterol levels frequently return to normal in eight to ten weeks. Mini meals also eliminate gas, bloating, indigestion and feeling distressingly full.

Mini meals can be conveniently dovetailed into most work schedules. You can eat one mini meal at breakfast, another at the mid-morning break, a third at lunch, a fourth in mid-afternoon, a fifth on arriving home from work, and three more during the evening. Hot meals are best eaten when at home where they can be rewarmed but you can carry a variety of fruits, salads, nuts and seeds to eat at work.

How Necessary Are Nutritional Supplements?

Whether or not you decide to reduce calorie intake, an abundant supply of vitamins, minerals and other nutrients is essential for optimal health and longevity. With the possible exception of Vitamin B_{12}, a diet of living foods provides an adequate supply of virtually every vitamin, mineral and enzyme needed by the human organism. Those of us who have lived for decades on the standard American diet frequently experience a decline in hydrochloric acid production by the stomach. As we age, this reduces our ability to absorb and utilize many minerals and vitamins.

Not surprisingly, a variety of studies by the USDA and other organizations have demonstrated that older people who continue to eat the standard American diet are frequently deficient in such key nutrients as Vitamins A, C, E and the B-complex, and in calcium, iron, magnesium and zinc, as well as in several trace elements.

Vitamania

Profit-motivated corporations and nutritional publications have siezed on these findings to promote the idea that the body can be put right by taking vitamins and other supplements that are conveniently available in health food stores.

We are told that by using supplements we can intervene in our own aging process. Megadoses of antioxidants will save us from the devastating effects of smoking. Growth hormones can supplement exercise. Various amino acids can prevent memory loss and senility.

To make it all easier, health food stores now carry special mixes of supplements to prevent memory loss, to make us smart, or to increase life expectancy, each with a convincing explanation of how it is all supposed to work. In reality, much of the data emphasizes isolated phenomena or minute trends, often based on questionable studies involving as few as half a dozen subjects. Much of the literature directly contradicts advice released by every major nutritional, scientific and health research organization.

To take megadoses of vitamins and other nutrients beneficially requires special knowledge. Taking megadoses of a single nutrient frequently increases need for other supplements in order to maintain balance. Any increase in one B-Vitamin, for instance, should be matched by a corresponding increase in the entire B-complex. There are hazards in taking excessive amounts of supplements like Vitamins A or B_6, or selenium. Again, many nutrients come in fillers, binders and capsules which, in large amounts, increase one's intake of undesirable dietary fat.

Thus, we should not be taken in by extravagant claims for "wonder" vitamins and nutrients. On the other hand, authentic studies have clearly shown that most Americans aged 50 and over could benefit from a good multi-vitamin mineral supplement each day.

Nutrients That Slow the Aging Process

Among key nutrients considered essential for slowing the aging process are Vitamins A, C, D, E, the entire B-complex (including Vitamin B_{12}), plus calcium, chromium, copper, iodine, iron, magnesium, manganese, phosphorous, potassium, selenium, and zinc. Most are supplied by a good multi-vitamin mineral supplement, though not always in the amounts necessary to meet the higher requirement of older people.

Anyone eating a diet high in living foods already has a plentiful supply of most essential nutrients. Whole grains, vegetables, legumes, nuts, seeds, fruits, fish, shellfish, skim milk and health food store items like brewer's yeast, raw wheat germ and lecithin granules should provide ample supplies of most anti-aging nutrients.

Supplements That Help Prevent Heart Disease

Nonetheless, people with a tendency toward cardiovascular disease, or those who already have it in any form, are often advised by nutritionists to increase their intake of anti-aging nutrients by supplementation and through sprinkling their food with wheat germ, brewer's yeast and lecithin—all rich in B Vitamins.

New information emerging from the frontiers of nutritional research is showing strong indications that coronary artery spasm is the actual cause of most angina pains and heart attacks. Artery spasm is often triggered by emotional stress but the underlying cause appears to be a deficiency of magnesium and potassium in the fluid in which the smooth muscles surrounding the coronary arteries are bathed. Tests in Germany in which heart disease patients were given supplements of magnesium orotate and potassium orotate—both available in health food stores in the United States—resulted in a mortality rate from heart disease only one-tenth that of a similar control group.

Supplements That Help Prevent Cancer

People with a tendency toward immune-system suppression or cancer are frequently advised to take supplements of antioxidants like Vitamins C and E, which prevent free radical damage by bonding with stray oxygen in the body. Considered vital for restoring the waning function of the thymus gland, and for absorbing free radicals, are Vitamin A and beta-carotene, Vitamins C, D and E together with calcium, selenium and zinc.

After menopause, women are especially prone to osteoporosis or bone loss. The risk of this condition can be diminished significantly through a program of daily exercise coupled with a high intake of calcium fortified with 400 I.U. daily of Vitamin D, and by not smoking. Most women over 45, especially those who eat animal protein, need 1,000 to 1,500 mgs of calcium daily to maintain calcium balance. Foods high in calcium are milk and dairy products, green leafy vegetables, and fish such as sardines and salmon. Lacking sufficient calcium from these sources, supplementary calcium should be taken, preferably in the form of calcium orotate. Vitamin D is supplied by fortified milk, fish liver oil, and by exposing the skin to the sun.

Retinoic acid, a form of Vitamin A—when taken with zinc—has greatly benefitted males with benign prostate enlargement, provided that a change-over is also made to a living foods diet coupled with a gradually increasing exercise program.

Supplements for Super Nutrition

Most nutritionists today recommend a total daily intake of vitamins and minerals—from both food sources and supplements—well in excess of the recommended daily allowance. However, the exact amount of each nutrient to be taken in supplement form depends on the amount already being supplied in one's diet. It is not possible to overdo the quantity of minerals and vitamins supplied in food. Certainly a daily vitamin-mineral supplement will do no harm. But need for additional supplementation must be judged by each individual, based on the ratio between complex carbohydrates already in the diet and by any tendency toward ccardiovascular disease, cancer or other chronic disease.

Within this framework, many modern nutritionists believe that we can safely take 5,000 I.U. daily of Vitamin A, a wide-spectrum B-complex formula that includes B_{12}, 1 or 2 grams daily of Vitamin C, 400 I.U. of Vitamin D, 400 mgs of Vitamin E, one gram of calcium, 400 mgs of magnesium, 50 micrograms of selenium and 15 mgs of zinc.

Supplements are best taken with meals and if you have a large assortment, they should be spread out over all three meals rather than all being taken together at a single meal.

In conclusion, diet and exercise work together to far exceed the benefits that either could achieve alone. Many of the benefits of exercise are lost for example, by continuing to eat a high-fat diet.

According to the best estimates, an 80-10-10 diet of living foods, combined with supplementation if needed and light eating—all integrated with daily exercise—can do more to promote a substantial increase in life expectancy than any other steps we could immediately take.

8

The Physical Approach
to Life Extension

Regular daily physical activity has been a way of life for virtually every person who has reached 100 in sound condition.

Alexander Leaf, a Harvard Medical School gerontologist, has described physical exercise as "the closest thing to an anti-aging pill." Scores of studies have provided incontestible proof that regular daily exercise such as walking, swimming or bicycling dramatically reduces risk of many degenerative diseases. In 1977, Arthur S. Leon, M.D., and Henry Blackburn, M.D., both of the University of Minnesota Medical School, published the result of a survey of all previous studies on the relationship between exercise and heart disease. They found a consistent pattern showing that physical inactivity and sedentary living are directly responsible for reduced cardiovascular and respiratory function and for diminished work capacity in older people. These diminished functions are not due to aging but to physical atrophy. From the results of the various studies, the two doctors concluded that exercise increases the diameter of the coronary arteries and stimulates growth of new collateral arteries when coronary arteries become blocked. Life expectancy is also increased independently of any cardiovascular benefit.

Other studies have demonstrated that regular exercise helps boost the efficiency of the immune system and reduces risk of cancer and auto-immune diseases. All research to date strongly indicates that regular exercise delays onset of most degenerative diseases and age-related dysfunctions. Once conditioned by exercise, the heart is much less prone to fibrillation and to sudden cardiac death. Bone density is maintained and the entire body becomes lean. Exercise, in fact, improves every quality associated with youth. Excess weight is burned off, and flexibility, balance, agility and coordination are frequently restored to youthful standards. Exercise increases strength, stamina, endurance and sexual vigor. Among the many positive side effects of exercise is that tension is replaced by relaxation, anxiety by contentment, and depression by optimism and aliveness. Most people who exercise regularly experience a psychological "high" that persists throughout the day.

LIFEX CONSTANT 5:   Exercise Regularly Every Day

Until the western world became mechanized, physical activity was a way of life for almost everyone. The need to walk everywhere, to housekeep without appliances, and to maintain large vegetable gardens kept older people at an acceptable level of fitness. Now we spend much of our lives sitting. We sit in front of TV sets, typewriters and computers; we sit in cars, golf carts and self-propelled lawnmowers; and we sit at meetings and in theaters and churches. The thousands of machines in use today have robbed us of the daily exercise on which the human body thrives. Active recreations, such as taking walks, have become a lost art in much of our culture. Today, most Americans are trapped in a world of physical inactivity in which we are unable to work off tension, burn off excess calories or exercise the heart and lungs.

Without daily exercise, our hearts become flabby and our arteries and muscles fade. By the mid 1950s, the American lifestyle had become so sedentary that heart disease was epidemic. Research by Dr. Kenneth Cooper and other cardiologists demonstrated that by exercising briskly for half an hour or more several times each week, we could restore a level of fitness essential for health and long life.

It was found, however, that only aerobic exercises would produce genuine fitness. An aerobic exercise is one which employs the large body muscles in a continuous, brisk and unbroken rhythm and which is sufficiently vigorous to increase oxygen uptake and cause panting. When maintained continuously for half an hour or more, aerobic exercises condition the heart, lungs and all other body systems while restoring an adequate supply of oxygen to every cell. Among the most beneficial aerobic exercises are running, jogging, brisk walking and race walking, swimming, brisk bicycling, cross-country skiing, skating, fast continuous dancing, rope skipping and such sports as basketball, squash, raquetball, soccer, handball and hockey. Also beneficial are such continuous rhythmic tasks as chopping, sawing, digging, paddling or rowing, or even hoeing and weeding—the type of manual labor on which our grandparents thrived.

Golf (with or without cart), baseball, softball, volleyball, doubles tennis, bowling and most forms of downhill skiing, provide fewer benefits.

A Powerful Catalyst to Revitalize the Body

Further research demonstrated that for maximum protection from cardiovascular disease, we should exercise at a pace sufficiently brisk to keep us in our "training effect" range for thirty minutes at a time on at least three occasions each week. A person's "training effect" range depends on age. You can easily calculate your personal "training effect" range by subtracting your age from 220. Ninety percent of the result equals your maximum pulse rate, which you should never exceed. Your "training effect" pulse rate lies between 70 and 85 percent of the result. (For a person aged 57, the calculation is 220 − 57 = 163. Ninety percent of 163 is 147, the maximum permissable pulse rate. Seventy percent of 163 is 114, and 85 percent is 139. Thus the "training effect" range lies between 114 and 139 beats per minute.)

Assuming you are 57, to obtain the benefits of the "training effect" you must exercise to maintain a pulse rate in the range of 114–139 for a minimum of thirty minutes at least three times each week.

To take your pulse while exercising, simply pause and count the beats for ten seconds and multiply by six. Begin by staying in your "training effect" range for just a few minutes. Although panting, you should be able to carry on a conversation without gasping. Then gradually work up to where your pulse remains in the "training effect" range for thirty minutes or more. At this point, you will experience a dramatic increase in heart and lung power, in oxygen uptake, and in increased energy, stamina and endurance. Your resting pulse rate will fall from the American average of 72 for men and 80 for women, to a more healthful 45 to 60 beats per minute. A resting pulse rate this low indicates that heart, lungs and arteries are in excellent condition. As you continue to exercise, the longer your pulse remains in the "training effect" range, the greater the benefit.

Ease Back into Shape

Few people can, or should, start right off by exercising in the "training effect" range. Most of us are so unaccustomed to exercise that we should begin at a low level of activity, such as walking, and increase speed and distance very gradually. In starting an exercise program, never exceed your capacity, never become fatigued, and avoid pushing yourself to the limit, at least until you are thoroughly conditioned.

Start out by walking one mile every day. If you cannot walk this far, go as far as you can without becoming fatigued. Ease into exercise very gradually. If you are badly out of shape, it may be weeks before you can walk a mile or more. But most healthy people can become capable walkers in just a few weeks.

Each day, walk a little farther and faster until you can cover a mile in fifteen minutes. At this point, walking will begin to produce some "training effect." Keep a record of how far and how fast you walk each day. After a month or so, many people find walking too easy and they are ready to jog.

Even if you never achieve "training effect," keep on walking. Studies have shown that LSD (long slow distance) exercising provides the same benefits as "training effect" by virtue of the distance alone. By walking six brisk miles in ninety-six minutes, for example, you can achieve the same benefits as by jogging for thirty minutes in your "training effect" range. The LSD principle can also be applied to most other forms of exercise.

The Hazards of Jogging

Jogging has become popular because it permits busy people to stay fit by cramming exercise into the shortest possible time. Yet it is not necessary to jog to become or stay fit. In fact, jogging is not desirable for most older people. The constant jolting of jogging, especially on hard surfaces, frequently causes sprains and pulled muscles. Over 40 percent of joggers eventually suffer from more serious injuries such as Achilles tendonitis, chondromalacia, plantar fascitis or heel spur, shin splints, neuroma and ankle neuritis. Such injuries may require lengthy recuperation with a possibility of permanent cartilage degeneration in hips, knees or back. Similar damage can result from rope skipping or from any exercise that involves continuous bouncing up and down.

Vitality Can Be Restored Without Jogging

Far preferable as exercises for life extension are aerobic activities such as walking, race walking, bicycling or swimming. These activities employ a smooth, fluid motion and can be enjoyed, free of injury, throughout one's life. "Training effect" can be reached just as readily by swimming, race walking, bicycling or by walking briskly uphill.

Because it frees the joints of almost any weight-bearing move- ment, swimming is perhaps the ideal way to exercise in the "training effect" range. This creates little risk of ever injuring a muscle, ligament or cartilage. Walking is another exercise that you can do safely at any age and maintain throughout life.

Should You Exercise?

Two questions frequently asked by sedentary, middle-aged people are: should I have a medical check-up before starting to exercise; and, am I too old to begin exercising?

Dr. George Sheehan, a pioneer of jogging, answered the first question by pointing out that the risk of not exercising far exceeds any risk involved in beginning a program of gradually increased daily exercise. However, if you are over 35, a steady smoker or drinker, or are overweight, you should check with a doctor before beginning any exercise program. The same caution applies if you have had, or suspect you may have, any form of cardiovascular disease, kidney problem, diabetes or any other chronic or degenerative disease.

Ask your doctor to give you a thallium test while running on a treadmill and, if necessary, a gated blood-pool study. These are more expensive than the stress EKG test normally used to reveal your maximum safe heartbeat rate, but EKG measurements often have a significant margin of error. Some people with heart disease are never detected while others with sound hearts may be falsely diagnosed as having heart disease.

If you do consult a doctor, make sure the doctor favors exercise. Consult only a physician who is slim and who exercises. Otherwise, a doctor prejudiced against exercise could give you biased and inaccurate advice.

Fortunately, most people can begin a program of brisk daily walking without consulting a physician.

When Are You Too Old to Exercise?

Scores of studies have provided proof that when people of mature years take up a structured exercise program, many signs of aging begin to disappear. The work of Herbert DeVries, director of exercise physiology at Andrus Gerontology Center, University of Southern California, has clearly demonstrated that popular ideas about people being too old to exercise are completely out of date. After conducting an exercise program for men and women averaging 70 years of age, Dr. DeVries found that much of their lost efficiency could be restored. At the end of forty-two weeks of regular exercise, the group had improved oxygen uptake by 29 percent, muscle strength by 12 percent, and vital capacity by 19 percent while they displayed significant loss of weight and reduction in blood pressure.

The result of these and other studies has led many gerontologists to recommend that Americans need *more* exercise after 50, not less. Most of us lead sedentary lives so that slowing down still further at 40, 50, or 60 can be a disastrous mistake. Yet the majority of us, in the mistaken belief that we may fall apart if we do anything strenuous, begin to avoid all vigorous activity on reaching middle age, including climbing hills and flights of stairs.

Although our physical capability does gradually slow with age, the process in fit, healthy people is barely perceptible. The annals are filled with records of long-lived people who somehow missed the news that they were too old to exercise and who went right on walking, running, swimming and skiing.

How to Tell If You Are Overdoing It

If you are aged between 30 and 55, a simple pulse test can show if you are overdoing exercise. After exercising, sit down and rest for sixty seconds. Then check your pulse. If it registers over 130 beats per minute, you are pushing yourself too hard. Reduce your speed and distance until your pulse registers closer to 100.

After resting a further five minutes, take your pulse again. A reading that exceeds 120 confirms that you are overdoing it. If after resting for ten full minutes, your pulse continues to register over 100, this is a final confirmation to reduce your speed and distance. For persons 55 and over, these figures should be gradually scaled down.

Other danger signals include pain and tightness in the chest with severe breathlessness, nausea, lightheadedness, dizziness or loss of muscular control. Should any of these occur during exercise, stop immediately and see a doctor.

Otherwise, you may continue to exercise safely and even take part in competitive sports. Marathon running, however, can be extremely stressful and may have a deleterious effect on the immune system and other body organs.

Several studies have shown that men and women who jog or swim moderate distances regularly derive almost equal cardiovascular benefits to those obtained by marathon runners. As the Framingham Heart Study has demonstrated (see Chapter 2) strict vegetarians actually have a lower risk of heart disease than marathon runners.

Scientific Proof That Exercise Prolongs Life

For over 4,000 years, humans have observed that fit, active people outlived those who were sedentary. But it was not until 1984 that scientific proof appeared to actually confirm that exercise *does* prolong life. A study of 17,000 Harvard alumnae by Dr. Ralph S. Paffenbarger, professor of epidemiology at Stanford University Medical School, revealed that men who expended 2,000 calories or more weekly on exercise showed a significant reduction in life-shortening diseases of the heart and arteries.

Conversely, the study showed that the most sedentary among the alumnae had a mortality rate almost twice as high as those who expended 2,000 calories or more on exercise each week. These conclusions were supported by a paralleling four-year study of 6,000 men and women made at the Institute for Aerobics Research in Dallas which concluded that sedentary people ran a 52 percent higher risk of developing hypertension than people who exercised regularly.

These studies, reported in the July 1984 issue of the Journal of the A.M.A. are regarded as a major breakthrough in linking increased exercise with longer life. While the studies showed that those who exercised most tended to live longest and experience the best health, they also demonstrated that even mild exercise like walking briskly four times a week, also contributed significantly to improving health and extending life.

How Diet Boosts the Benefits of Exercise

As discussed in Chapter 2, the physical risk of heart disease is best assessed by dividing the cholesterol level by the HDL level. The lower the cholesterol level and the higher the HDL level, the more favorable is the prognosis for heart disease risk. Serum cholesterol level can be lowered only by reducing dietary fat. The level of HDL in the bloodstream can be increased only by exercise.

Exercise alone primarily reduces risk of heart disease by raising the HDL level. But when a program of regular aerobic exercise is combined with a lean and low-fat diet (Lifex Constants 3 and 4), the result is a powerful combination that works to dramatically reduce risk of cardiovascular and other degenerative diseases.

So effective is this combination that some cardiologists refer to it as the "exercise-diet equation" (aerobic exercise + lean, low-fat diet = low heart disease risk). Thus, the benefits of exercise are more than doubled when a lean, low-fat diet is also included.

Other Exercises

How effective are other types of exercise like weight-lifting, calisthenics or stretching exercises? Weight-training, which consists of many brisk repetitions of traditional weight-lifting exercises while using much lighter weights, can tone up the entire body while also providing some aerobic benefit. Provided that cartilage-damaging exercises like deep knee-bends and full sit-ups are omitted, calisthenics can have the same effect.

For those who enjoy group exercise to music, health spas and exercise classes can also be worthwhile.

Exercises which lock knee or elbow should be strictly avoided due to the high risk of cartilage injury. To restore youthful flexibility, yoga postures or "asanas" are recommended. A brief warm-up that includes a few basic stretches should precede any exercise period in order to minimize risk of muscle pulls or sprains.

Once in condition, exercise in every way you can. Walk up flights of stairs instead of taking the elevator. Walk all or part way to and from work. Use every opportunity to increase the amount of movement and strenuous effort in your life.

Exercising Outdoors Is Better

Exercise outdoors whenever you can. John N. Ott—a photographic inventor and an expert in optics—is among many authorities who emphasize the need to spend more time outdoors so that we orient ourselves to nature. Exposing the eyes regularly to full-spectrum sunlight benefits both the eyes and the entire body, Ott explains. Many of us, by contrast, spend most of our time indoors under artificial light, a combination which encourages numerous diseases.

Sunbathing

Equally unwise, however, is excessive exposure to solar radiation. A brief fifteen-minute sunbath when the sun is not higher than 45° above the horizon produces a pleasing light tan and stimulates production of Vitamin D.

Recent discoveries have revealed that lying out in the midday sun acquiring a deep copper tan can have a disastrous long-term effect on health and longevity. To begin with, bombardment of the skin by ultra-violet light sets off a free-radical chain reaction that destroys the flexibility and elasticity of the skin, causing it to age prematurely. Tanning, which is actually the skin's response to photo-toxic injury, may eventually lead to a variety of skin disorders.

Solar radiation can create severe suppression of the immune system. Since 10 percent of the blood is always in the skin, the entire blood supply is subject to a form of immune suppression called photo-immunology whenever we expose our skin to the sun for extended periods.

Following over-exposure to the sun, the immune system becomes severely depressed for up to fifteen days or more. During this time, infections like cold sores, or auto-immune conditions like purpura, are able to develop. A number of scientists engaged in photo-immunology research believe that several types of cancer could develop after prolonged exposure to the sun.

LIFEX CONSTANT 6:   Mobilize a Store of Physical Energy

Healthy, long-lived people have such boundless energy that they seldom suffer from the middle-aged weariness and fatigue that seem to plague most Americans.

The Dynamics of Fatigue

Weariness and fatigue are caused by a number of habits including unresolved stress, a diet high in fats and refined carbohydrates, indulgence in stimulants, or insufficient exercise.

Working in different ways, either separately or in combination, these factors reduce the oxygen and glucose carried by the bloodstream to tissue, brain and muscle cells. Without sufficient oxygen, the muscles are unable to oxidize glucose efficiently, the body's principal form of fuel. Without sufficient oxygen, the muscles become clogged with lactic acid, a form of residual ash left over from the burning of glucose. It is through this mechanical process— created by dietary fat—that weariness and fatigue are produced. (Fish body oils are believed to be the only fat which do not contribute to fatigue.)

Glucose, the energy which fuels our muscles, is derived primarily from carbohydrates such as starchy vegetables and grains. The process of converting food into energy involves almost every stage in the entire metabolism of the human organism. For this complex process to begin, the body must first be challenged by exercise. In response to any type of rhythmic exercise, the body's entire metabolic process is set in motion and each stage then keeps producing energy for several hours afterward.

How to Mobilize Energy

A body unused to exercising tires at the slightest effort. We can eat high-energy food but if we are inactive, we will always feel weary and tired. To generate energy, we must exercise first. Only by exercising can we challenge the body's metabolism to begin mobilizing energy.

If, for example, you wish to have the energy to walk ten miles without fatigue, you must first challenge the body by walking one mile. In response to the challenge of having walked one mile, the body will mobilize sufficient energy to walk one mile on the following day plus a margin for extra distance. If, each day, we increase the distance we walk by one mile, in just ten days we can mobilize all the energy we need to keep on walking ten miles every day without effort or fatigue.

Simply by practicing Lifex Constants 3 and 5—eating a low-fat diet and exercising regularly—middle-aged fatigue and weariness will begin to disappear. To ensure that this happens, however, we must also practice Lifex Constant 1 by minimizing dependence on medical care (including avoidance of drugs of all types); Lifex Constant 2, by eliminating all stimulants; and Lifex Constants 11, 12 and 13, through which we can learn to resolve stress in non-harmful ways.

In practice, much fatigue is also created by muscular tension resulting from unresolved stress. The unrelieved tension continually burns energy, leaving the body weary and depleted. Here again, the best antidote is Lifex Constant 5: exercise regularly every day. Half an hour of brisk aerobic exercise will transform the most stubborn level of stress and tension into a feeling of relaxed calm.

Beat the Fatigue Slump

Other important steps in ending weariness and fatigue are to strictly avoid all junk food, including any product containing sugar and white flour, caffeine, nicotine or alcohol. All these provide a swift flush of energy that sends the blood sugar level soaring. Then as the nutrient supply is quickly exhausted, blood sugar levels come crashing down again. Almost all fatigue coincides with a low blood-sugar level.

LIFEX CONSTANT 7:   Avoid Becoming Tired or Fatigued

It is natural to feel tired and sleepy by bedtime, but if you feel tired earlier, go to bed. Do not wait until your usual bedtime. In his book, *The Long-Lived of Soviet Georgia,* Dr. G.Z. Pitzkhelauri points out that almost all long-lived people in the Soviet Caucasus take a regular daily period of relaxation.

If circumstances are such that you do become tired and exhausted, try to limit it to a single day. Avoid becoming weary and fatigued on two consecutive days or for any longer period.

One of the best ways to relax is to lie down in a quiet place. Then, one by one, tense each muscle in the body as tightly as you can, hold for six seconds and release. Tense and release, in turn, each arm, each leg, the abdomen muscles, the chest and shoulders, and the neck and facial muscles. Then imagine that your hands are tingling and becoming heavy and warm. Say to yourself, "My hands feel heavy and warm. Warmth is flowing into my hands. My hands are heavy and tingling with warmth."

As you repeat these phrases slowly and silently to yourself, your hands will become warm and heavy.

Your central nervous system has relaxed the smooth muscles that constrict arteries in your hands, allowing more blood to flow into your hands to warm them. This effect gradually generalizes through every artery in your body, including your coronary arteries. As it does, you will reach a deep level of relaxation that will restore and rejuvenate your body and mind.

LIFEX CONSTANT 8:   Maintain Recommended Body Weight

Few, if any, long-lived people are overweight. Studies made in both the U.S. and the U.S.S.R. have all shown a relationship between being lean and living longer. The studies indicate that people who are significantly overweight, or whose weight has increased by ten pounds or more since age 21, lose two or more years from their life expectancy. Yet according to the Metropolitan Life Insurance Company's 1983 height and weight charts, 45 percent of American men and 33 percent of American women are overweight.

As a result, weight loss has become a major industry in America. Shelves in bookstores, health food shops and supermarkets are crammed with weight-loss books that promise to melt away surplus pounds in a matter of days. Some books promise rapid weight loss without either physical exercise or will-power. Yet omission of these two essential requirements guarantees that any weight-loss plan will fail.

Diets That Do Not Work

Many weight-loss books describe fad diets that are high in fat and animal protein and are nutritionally unsound in numerous other ways. Millions of overweight Americans buy one new diet book after another. With each new book, they gain the motivation to lose a few pounds. But after a few weeks, they fail to stay with their new diet and their weight goes soaring up again.

People who alternatively diet and then eat excessively, and whose weight keeps fluctuating, are at a higher risk of disease than those who are constantly overweight.

Fad diets fail because they are not holistic. Modern weight-loss experts have discovered that each person has a setpoint that controls the amount of body fat like a thermostat controls heat. Lean people have a low setpoint while in overweight people, the setpoint is high. When we strive to lose weight with a high setpoint, the body stubbornly resists in order to preserve its store of body fat. Diets that deprive us of our normal calorie input make us irritable and lacking in energy. Yet bookstores, magazines and the weekly tabloids are constantly filled with diet plans based on the assumption that we can lose weight by reducing our calorie input alone.

The only way to lose weight permanently is to lower your setpoint for body fat. This setpoint can be lowered only by a Whole Person approach. Overeaters Anonymous, a weight-loss support group, considers compulsive eating to be a physical, emotional and even spiritual dysfunction that can be reversed only through a holistic approach.

Millions of Americans, especially women, turn to food for relief when under stress. Since infancy, most of us have associated food with warmth, security and love. Hence, compulsive eating has become a tranquilizer and the drug of choice for millions of overstressed people. As we eat compulsively and put on weight, the cells in our tissues constantly signal our body-fat setpoint to demand more food, particularly foods rich in fat and refined carbohydrates. Anyone with a surplus of fat cells is constantly under pressure to supply these cells with more and more fat by eating increasing amounts of food.

How to Break the Vicious Cycle

This vicious metabolic circle can be broken only by gradually lowering the setpoint through a holistic combination of regular daily aerobic exercise and the 80-10-10 way of eating. The complex carbohydrate diet allows us to continue eating the food we want, while the exercise reduces hunger pangs, burns off excess weight, and overcomes the stress-related emotions that motivate compulsive eating. The result is that our fat setpoint gradually falls back to normal and our weight returns to normal. For as long as we stay with the 80-10-10 eating plan, and continue to exercise adequately, our weight will remain permanently at the normal level.

Plan to begin a program of gradually increasing exercise on the same day that you start your diet transformation. You will not experience hunger because you can eat almost unlimited amounts of complex carbohydrate foods without gaining weight.

To improve results, omit all avocadoes, nuts and seeds until your weight is back to normal. You can help speed weight loss, and later maintain your normal weight, by breaking up your standard meals into smaller and more frequent mini meals (see Lifex Constant 4). Supervised tests have proven that people who switch to a mini-meal routine frequently lose one to two pounds per week without reducing calorie intake.

It also helps to consume the majority of your daily calorie intake before eleven in the morning. Naturally, all this assumes that you also abstain from alcohol, whole milk or other fattening beverages.

What Is Your Ideal Weight?

For the first time in twenty-four years, the Metropolitan Insurance Company revised its height-weight charts in 1983. Recommended weights rose three to ten pounds for women and two to thirteen pounds for men. The new tables are not listed as "desirable" weights but represent the weights at which 4.2 million life insurance policy holders lived longest in recent years. The new tables reveal that people are living longer at higher weights.

But experts in organizations such as the American Heart Association and the National Institutes of Health have suggested that people are not actually living longer because of higher weights. They believe that people are living longer because upgraded lifestyle habits such as eating less fat, exercising and non-smoking have offset the effects of increased weight.

Meanwhile, the American Heart Association urges Americans to follow the older height–weight tables published in 1959. Dr. W. Virgil Brown, chairman of the AHA's nutrition committee, recently pointed out that "heart disease increases as body weight increases. And few health problems are improved by gaining weight." Dr. Brown's sentiments were echoed by Dr. Artemis Simopoulos of the National Institutes of Health, who said of the new tables that "the most important message is that the desirable weight is still below average. And people with below average weight still generally live longer."

Based on findings by the California State Health Department and the American Society of Actuaries, the optimum weight for long life is approximately 3 percent below the "desirable" weights in Metropolitan's 1959 tables. Thus, for maximum life extension, a man six feet tall with a medium frame would have an ideal weight of 144 to 157 pounds in indoor clothing (compared with 148 to 162 pounds in Metropolitan's 1959 tables and 157 to 170 pounds in their 1983 tables). Reducing weight more than 3 percent below levels in Metropolitan's 1959 tables is not recommended and may actually shorten life.

How to Regain a Slim, Youthful Figure

A few simple facts of physics explain why the 80-10-10 way of eating (see Chapter 7, "Eating the 80-10-10 Way"), coupled with a regular aerobic exercise, works unfailingly to restore weight to normal. One food-calorie contains the heat required to raise one kilogram of water one degree Centigrade. On this basis, one pound of body fat contains the equivalent of 3,500 stored food calories.

To maintain body metabolism requires a dietary intake of approximately 15 calories per day per pound of body weight at age 35. Thus, a 160-pound man requires roughly 2,400 calories per day from food and drink to maintain normal weight. Per gram, fat contains 9.3 calories, protein or refined carbohydrate 4.1 calories and complex carbohydrates only 2.75. As we increase consumption of complex carbohydrates, the fewer calories we absorb and the more fiber we take in. Fiber bulks up the stomach and intestines and keeps us feeling full. Complex carbohydrates are the main ingredients of the 80-10-10 way of eating. By eating 100 fewer calories per day, in thirty-five days you will eliminate one pound of fat. If you also burn up 100 calories per day through exercise, in thirty-five days you will also lose one pound of fat.

Melt Away Pounds with Exercise

Innumerable tests have demonstrated that increased exercise does not result in increased hunger. Hence, the best way to accelerate weight loss is to exercise more vigorously. While walking burns up only 300 calories per hour, chopping and sawing wood consume 450 calories, brisk bicycling uses 500 calories, jogging, ski-touring or swimming the crawl require 600 calories, and rowing takes 675 calories per hour.

Weight cannot be lost and kept off permanently unless exercise is included in the program together with diet. In a study at Kansas State University, Dr. William Z. Zuti, director of exercise physiology, found that women who dieted to lose weight lost both fat and lean tissue while women who exercised lost only fat. Loss of lean tissue is undesirable. Dr. Zuti concluded that exercising as you diet is by far the healthiest way to lose weight.

Through a program based on exercise plus the 80-10-10 eating plan, both your body-fat setpoint and your actual body weight will gradually drop to normal. Your weight will then stabilize at its optimal level. You may then restore such fatty complex carbohydrates as avocadoes, nuts and seeds. If you begin eating vegetable oils, animal fats or refined carbohydrates, your weight is likely to begin increasing once more.

LIFEX CONSTANT 9:   Maintain an Erect Posture

At any age, a slouching posture leads to shallow breathing, a reduced intake of oxygen, a distended abdomen that inhibits the function of vital organs, increased tension in the skeletal muscles, and sometimes a depressed mood and outlook. Such a condition causes a variety of dysfunctions from arthritis to lower back pain.

The older we are and the less we exercise, the greater the tendency is to slouch. Thus, the older we are, the greater our need to stand straight and erect once again. In most cases, poor posture can be quite easily corrected. Women should begin by discarding high-heeled shoes, which are responsible for a multitude of postural problems.

The worst way to try to improve your carriage is to consciously make yourself erect by holding the military stance. You cannot continue to hold your tummy in, chest out and head upright for very long without discomfort.

Instead, start by constantly recalling the three keys to good posture.

1.   Tilt your pelvis back.

2.   Lift your chest.

3.   Begin every movement by raising your head and stretching your spine upward.

All that is necessary is to visualize these factors in your mind. Your muscles will then move subconsciously to express the erect, youthful carriage you are visualizing.

Tilting your pelvis back results in contracting your abdomen or tucking in your tummy. Do not try to use your muscles to do it consciously. Simply visualize your pelvis tilted back.

Your posture will improve rapidly if you can remember to begin every body movement by raising your head up and away from the body. This is the primary principle behind the famous Alexander Technique for natural movement and poise. When you walk upstairs, for example, let your head lead the body in moving upward and forward. As you do, your spine will lengthen and your posture will become relaxed and erect.

A good tip when walking is to imagine you are hanging suspended from a hook in the top of your head. Picture your entire body relaxed and hanging loose and straight like a puppet on a string. Immediately, you will find you are walking straight and tall with a long, flowing stride.

Keep the back straight when sitting or bending. Instead of curving the spine as you bend over, bend from the hips and keep the back straight.

After a week or two, this will become a constant habit. Your new, erect posture will make you feel good about yourself. Your self-image will improve, your lung capacity will increase, and you will look taller and slimmer.

LIFEX CONSTANT 10:   Live in a Healthy Environment

It is not necessary to live in Shangri-La to live long and healthfully. Your chances for health and long life in the United States are among the best, provided you live in an environment that nurtures wellness and longevity.

Until recent years, statistics showed that Americans lived longest in small, rural towns and on farms. But latest trends are revealing that the mechanization and widespread use of toxic pesticides have made farming a high-risk occupation. Lack of fresh fruits, vegetables and grains in small towns, coupled with a reluctance of most small town residents to exercise, is cutting down their traditional longevity lead.

However, big cities remain as hostile to human life as ever. Temperature inversion in Denver, Los Angeles, New York and other metropolitan centers increases risk of pulmonary and cardiac diseases. The noise, overcrowding, high crime rate, and fast pace are all stressful.

As a result, life expectancy is increasing in suburban areas throughout the country and in small resorts and college towns with populations of less than 100,000. Quiet, spacious, verdant suburbs and smaller unpolluted cities, now appear to offer America's most nurturing environments for health and long life.

The Healthiest Places to Live

Because suburbs and small towns are home to the most affluent and highly educated groups, every kind of service and facility that benefits human health are available. They are well supplied with natural food stores and grainaries. Bicycle travel is usually safe and practical. There are jogging and hiking trails and numerous parks. In college towns, and frequently elsewhere, there is a steady succession of stimulating cultural events and lectures as well as numerous opportunities to study everything from art to zen.

The most nurturing environment is a compromise between living in quiet, stress-free suburbs, and urban areas.

Higher Is Healthier

Among geographic variables, elevation appears to have the greatest effect on health. Surveys show that throughout the world, people who live in mountain villages have fewer heart attacks. If they do suffer heart attacks, they are less likely to die than people who live in flat, urban environments. Also, throughout the world, the higher the elevation, the lower the incidence of cancer and cardiovascular disease.

This discovery, made only in recent years, has led cardiologists to send their patients to altitudes of six or seven thousand feet to recover. The University of Colorado Health Services at Denver explains that after a few weeks at higher altitude, our red blood-cell count increases. The result is that the quantity of blood pumped by the heart is cut by as much as 20 percent. This eases the burden on the heart.

Initially, the heart must work harder at higher elevations. But after a few weeks, as red blood cells multiply, its task is eased. Once you have become acclimatized, living at an altitude of five to seven thousand feet decreases risk of heart attack.

This finding concurs with the observation that many long-lived societies—such as the hill farmers of Hunza, Vilcabamba and Abkhasia—lead active lives at elevations of four to seven thousand feet.

America's Most Salubrious Region

North America sustains many dry, sunny areas with elevations of five to seven thousand feet. Such states are Colorado, Utah, Northern Arizona and New Mexico, and also the neighboring plateau of Mexico. Within this area are such liveable towns as Boulder, Colorado; Cedar City, Utah; Prescott, Arizona; and Santa Fe, New Mexico, as well as San Miguel de Allende and the Lake Chapala area in Mexico.

Throughout this vast region, climate and topography closely resemble those of Hunza, Vilcabamba and Abkhasia. But to benefit from living in these areas we must also approximate the active lifestyles and low-fat diet of the hill farmers of Hunza, Vilcabamba and Abkhasia. We must walk vigorously up and down the many hills; we must swim, bicycle, ski cross-country and exercise our minds and bodies in every possible way.

Wherever we choose to live, the climate and environment should permit us to exercise outdoors throughout the year. There should be a minimum of pollution and stress from noise or traffic.

9

The Psychological Approach to Life Extension

Stress is the primary factor which influences our health. Stress arises from our psychological attitudes, values and beliefs. Nothing ages us faster than guilt, resentment, anger, worry, and fear.

Through the Lifex Constants in this chapter, we learn how long-lived people are able to transform their attitudes, beliefs and values so that destructive stress is controlled.

LIFEX CONSTANT 11: Adopt a Flexible Attitude and Accept Necessary Change

Several years ago, Dr. Robert W. Samp of the University of Wisconsin studied the lifestyle profiles of one thousand people aged over 75, including 130 centenarians. He compared their lifestyle habits with those of a control group of one thousand people aged 54–74, many of whom suffered from degenerative diseases. Dr. Samp found that the two key constants which occurred time and again in the longevous group were moderation and flexibility.

The ability to be flexible and to adapt to change is one of the strongest keys to long life. Dr. Samp found that healthful, long-lived people are able to accept change without emotional damage. They have learned to respond to stress in a calm, serene way. They do not repress emotions, but they remain calm and untouched by the chaos around them.

Throughout the world, healthy, long-lived people have this ability to flow with life's adversities. Out of this ability emerges a strong resilience that permits them to rebound unharmed, time and again, from the damaging effects of stress. Take the case of Lynn and Lydia Wells of Denniston, Kentucky. The long lives of this couple had been jolted no less than six times—five times by tragic accidents which killed five of their sons and a sixth time when their house burned down. Yet in every case they were able to rebound and begin life again. Then tragedy struck once more. When Lynn was 96 and Lydia 94, their house burned down a second time and they lost all their possessions. Even at that age, the couple still possessed the resilience to spring back. A short time later, the Wells were living on their own once more in a new mobile home.

Escape Stress

The Stress Theory describes aging as the cumulative total of all the stress that occurs in a lifetime. Even flexible people who can transform stress into non-stress fare better when their lives are subject to fewer changes. For stress is anything which makes it difficult to adapt to life's changes. Any kind of change can, therefore, be stressful.

Dr. Dmitri Chebotarev, a Russian gerontologist, who studied the long-lived peoples of the Soviet Caucasus, concluded that the steady uninterrupted rhythm of nature is responsible for their health and longevity. Throughout their lives, these country dwellers rise and go to bed at the same time; they do the same, satisfying work; and they avoid most of the pressures and stressful changes of life in industrialized nations.

A study by Dr. Francis D. Glamser of the Center for Studies in Aging at North Texas State University found similar conditions among long-term convicts in American prisons. Prisoners who have spent long years living the same orderly, routine prison life, with a minimum of change, maintain the appearance, posture and vigor of younger people. Several men and women in jails in the United States have reached age 100 in a healthful condition. Dr. Glamser concluded that prisoners age 30 percent more slowly, both physically and mentally, than people outside prison, primarily because they are not subject to multiple stressful changes.

Other surveys have shown that people who make frequent changes in life and who often move and change friends, spouses, jobs or residences frequently, lose two or more years from their life expectancy. Even relatively pleasant events such as marriage, the addition of a child to a family, or travel can be stressful. Jet lag, for example, places increasing demands on the heart and arteries and has triggered thousands of heart attacks.

From all this information, gerontologists have defined two key lifestyle factors through which we can significantly extend life. The first is to lead an orderly life in which unnecessary and disturbing change is minimized. The second is to minimize stress by becoming more flexible and learning to adapt freely to change.

Avoid Wrenching Change

Exactly how we can minimize unnecessary and disturbing change in our lives is something each of us must answer for ourselves. We can, for instance, examine our daily lives and cut down on such stressful activities as freeway driving and commuting. We should get up at the same time every morning, including weekends, and go to bed when we feel tired. Without destroying opportunities for serendipity and spontaneity, we should organize as much of our daily lives as we can on a stress-free basis.

Meanwhile, we can make a giant step toward minimizing stress by becoming more flexible and learning to adapt to change. To do so, we must first realize that stress does not actually arise from the changes and events in our lives. Life events and changes are neutral. It is how we perceive and react to an event that creates stress. Frequently, we react out of fear of loss and insufficiency.

Jones and Smith, for example, are both laid off from their jobs on a Detroit production line. Jones sees his layoff as a total disaster. He believes that no other job will ever materialize and he fears losing his home and car through inability to maintain payments. Smith, in contrast, views his layoff as a welcome relief from a boring, monotonous job. He plans to use his enforced leisure to train for a more interesting and rewarding job in the computer field.

Jones felt threatened because he believed in a me-versus-them world in which there were too few jobs, homes, cars and money to go around and that one person could win only if another loses. Smith's beliefs were positive and optimistic. Through them, he viewed the world as a friendly place with enough for us all to be able to win.

It is our dogmatic beliefs and learned responses to stressful situations that make us rigid and unable to adapt to changes. Modern life is filled with potentially stressful situations that make us rigid and unable to adapt to changes. Modern life is filled with potentially stressful situations to which we must constantly adapt. Being too rigid and too inflexible to flow with life's events creates inner conflicts. Reduce stress by accepting situations in life that are beyond our power to change. Instead of rigidly fighting adversities, we must accept those which cannot be prevented. Through these changed beliefs, events that we now regard as stressful can be transformed into challenging new opportunities.

How to Handle Stress Creatively

Stress can be also offset through a series of coping mechanisms. First and foremost is regular daily aerobic exercise (see Lifex Constant 5). Studies by

Dr. Herbert DeVries and others have demonstrated conclusively that a brisk daily walk is a splendid natural tranquilizer. Swimming, bicycling, jogging or any other type of rhythmic exercise is a proven antidote to stress.

When you are faced with a stressful situation, and feel yourself about to become angry and tense, try this four-stage coping technique. First: stop everything completely. Second: do absolutely nothing. Third: take twelve long, slow, deep breaths. Fourth: relax–shrug your shoulders, roll your neck and relax your eyes, facial muscles and eyelids. As you do, imagine you are relaxing at your favorite beach on a warm, summer day. By the time you have gone through this routine, the situation will seem much less threatening. You can deliberately choose to adopt a flexible attitude and to flow along with the problem instead of resisting it.

Psychologists recommend that much stress can be transformed into non-stress by simply changing our beliefs about hostility, resentment and competing.

Hostility may be the most dangerous element in the Type A personality. Dr. Redford B. Williams of Duke University studied the lives of 255 physicians who had taken a personality inventory as medical students. He found that over the next twenty-five years, those with the highest hostility scores had a death rate of 14 percent versus only 2.5 percent among those with the lowest hostility scores. Among the hostile group, heart disease was five times as common. Williams defined hostility as an attitude of distrust and dislike of people that often triggers anger. We can extend our lives by transforming our distrust and dislike of people into an attitude of acceptance, friendliness and love.

Resentment builds to a dangerous level when you do not forgive others. People who say, "I will never forgive _____," are expressing a rigid belief that can affect their health. You can overcome this attitude by forgiving everyone you believe may have caused you harm.

Competing with others can keep us permanently drained of energy. Instead, compete with excellence, not with other people. Learn to do something well, then attempt to beat your own best efforts. Be willing to share your knowledge with others.

You can make your attitude even more flexible through another four-step technique. First: Admit to yourself that you are fearful of change. Most of us fear change because of a possible loss of our security or lifestyle. We are not afraid of the loss itself, but of how we are going to cope with that loss. Second: Practice meeting changes by making small, new changes in your life each week. Plan to exchange some of your familiar routines for new ones.

For instance, you might decide to take a walk during your lunch break instead of eating in your office. Third: Put these new changes into practice. Fourth: Evaluate how successfully you have adapted to each change.

Gradually, as you become more flexible, you can adapt to larger changes without incurring stress. Eventually, you may become so flexible that you actually welcome change.

Anti-Stress Technologies That Work

You can accept stress more readily by conquering your fear of the unknown. If you must face an upcoming change, think of the most stressful thing that could happen and ask yourself how bad it would really be. Visualize the lifestyle adjustments you would have to make to adapt, and practice living these in your imagination. Previewing stress in your imagination makes you much less vulnerable when you actually encounter a stressful change.

You can also minimize stress by practicing a yoga technique called witnessing. Instead of reacting to a potentially stressful event, you simply observe it and witness it dispassionately without reacting. If you are upset by a loud motorcycle exhaust, for instance, the next time you hear one, simply relax and tell yourself, "I am witnessing the sound of a motorcycle exhaust. I have no emotional reaction at all." In this way, you can rapidly desensitize yourself to an upsetting stimuli.

Meditation is another technique through which your mind can become calm and serene. To meditate, simply sit upright in a quiet place where you will not be disturbed. Relax and begin to breathe slowly and deeply. Look quietly at your surroundings and witness them. Witness and observe each object you can see without experiencing any reaction. Then close your eyes.

As you inhale, visualize the figure "1." As you exhale, open your eyes and silently chant "Om." On the following inhalation, close your eyes and visualize the figure "2"; then exhale as you open your eyes and silently chant "Om." With each inhalation, visualize a consecutive figure until you finally reach 100. At that point, your mind should be quiet and serene.

Close your eyes and begin to witness the thoughts that flow through your mind. View each thought as a friendly experience. As you witness each thought, it will disappear. Soon, your mind will become totally quiet and free of thoughts. At that point, begin to witness your breathing while still being aware of any passing thoughts.

Meditate once or twice daily for twenty or thirty minutes. Studies have confirmed that meditation lowers blood pressure and risk of heart disease.

We cannot change our emotions, but we *can* change our thoughts. A negative thought precedes every negative emotion. Anger cannot occur unless preceded by an angry thought. Thus, whenever you recognize a thought as provoking anger, envy, resentment, fear or hostility, immediately replace it with a thought of something you enjoy. By eliminating stressful thoughts, we can eliminate harmful emotions.

LIFEX CONSTANT 12:   Cultivate an Optimistic Outlook

At age 109, Walter Jones was still recently touring America lecturing on health. His advice was that "worrying is a waste of time." Jones recommended that to avoid worry, we simply tune in to the good things in life and forget the bad.

Jones is not alone in his views. Records show that healthy, long-lived people spend little time in worrying. They are concerned about problems but they take their problems in stride. If they are able to solve a problem, they do so. If they cannot, they accept the problem. They rarely worry about anything that is beyond their control.

Like Walter Jones, longevous people overcome fear and worry by realizing that most things we fear and worry about never happen. Even if a fear did materialize, it is seldom likely to be catastrophic.

Through cultivating a flexible attitude, healthy well-adjusted people of any age are confident that whatever happens, they can take it in stride and adjust readily to the new circumstance. Well-adjusted people are resourceful creatures with tremendous ability to adapt to changing conditions. With a flexible attitude, we can accept any kind of change and adapt to it without stress.

Many long-lived people maintain an optimistic outlook. As a result, problems and failures are transformed into new and exciting opportunities. When one door closes, another door usually opens. Should a feared event occur, invariably it opens another door to something new, better and more profitable. One retired man who worried about his home being burglarized while he was away, found eventually that his home had been broken into. In response, he launched a home security service that now supplies him with a generous income.

LIFEX CONSTANT 13:   Slow Down. Avoid Stress. Live in the Present Moment

Liberating oneself from time schedule pressure is an art. We can free ourselves from time urgency by slowing down, by doing only one thing at a time, and by living in the present instead of in the past or future.

Time-pressure stress, one of the most destructive traits in the Type A personality, occurs when we try to do too many activities in too little time. To maintain a round of busy schedules means we must constantly watch the clock and be rigidly punctual. The typical Type A person cannot tolerate an unfinished job. The pressure is intensified further because most Type A's are also perfectionists. Through believing that only they can do a job satisfactorily, they fail to delegate work to subordinates and insist on doing it all themselves.

Longevous people, who are almost always well-adjusted Type B's, have invariably mastered the art of serenity. Frequently, they are able to accomplish as much as the Type A person, but their lives are geared to a slower, more leisurely pace.

How can we escape the destructive pressure of deadlines and schedules that crowd in from every side? Through incorporating relaxed traits into your personal lifestyle, you can frequently accomplish a great deal without the killing pace.

By incorporating the following good health habits into your life, you will begin to free yourself from time-pressure stress.

• **Slow Down.** Deliberately slow down so that you eat, work, play and talk at a relaxed, leisurely pace. Actively cultivate relaxation and patience. Schedule frequent breaks each day for fun and socializing.

• **Schedule Time Alone Each Day.** Time-pressure stress always involves other people. Learn to enjoy spending some time each day by yourself without feeling lonely. Free of involvement with others, you immediately discover time for renewal. You are free to do what you most enjoy, think anything you wish, walk alone in the country, or renew yourself by writing, painting, or playing an instrument.

• **Refuse to Be Rigidly Punctual.** Deliberately avoid being right on time. Set appointments for a flexible time such as "around three o'clock." Give yourself ample time to reach your next appointment and to prepare for it.

Avoid any self-imposed deadlines or schedules. Let what you cannot do today wait until tomorrow or another day.

Without being aggressive, become quite assertive about saying "No" to people who place demands on your time. Turn down any request for non-essential community or volunteer work that might create pressure in your life. Concentrate only on activities through which you make a genuine contribution. Do not be afraid of offending people. You do not need the approval of everyone all of the time. Your health is more important than trying to please everybody.

• **Learn to Live with Unfinished Jobs.** Having unfinished jobs on hand should not be disturbing. If you cannot complete a job today, accept that you can carry on with it tomorrow or next week. To achieve serenity, we must be willing to live with uncompleted jobs. So relax and enjoy life instead of worrying about how to complete every unfinished task. In just a short time, you will become completely comfortable with having unfinished jobs around and you will no longer experience any sense of time urgency to get everything completed.

• **Minimize Waiting Time.** You can create more time in your life by setting up activities like shopping, going to the bank or dentist, so that you minimize having to wait. Stores are least crowded right after opening time on weekdays while supermarkets are often quite empty late in the evening. Avoid banking during peak business hours. You can avoid waiting in line by using twenty-four-hour computer tellers. To minimize waiting at doctor or dentist offices, book the first slot after opening in the morning or after lunch.

• **Make Your Activities Monophasic.** Doing only one thing at a time, (known as monophasic activity as compared to polyphasic activity) forces you to slow down. Instead of gulping breakfast while you read the paper, you are free to become absorbed in tasting your breakfast. As a result, you will be more relaxed.

• **Live in the Present.** Many longevous people learned early in life to stop feeling guilty about the past and to stop worrying about the future. They learned instead to live in the present moment and to enjoy it to the fullest. While it is necessary to give some thought to the future, well-adjusted Type B's spend little time regretting what they did in the past or worrying about what the future may bring.

Most of us anticipate being happier in the future: when the children leave home, when vacation time arrives, or when we retire. But when that time actually arrives, we find we are no happier than before. To assume that we can be happier in the future is simply setting ourselves up for disappointments. The only time we can experience happiness is in the present.

Through having learned to maximize enjoyment of the present, longevous people are seldom bored. To experience life fully, we should begin to see, smell, touch and feel everything around us. Concentrate on what you are doing at this moment. In this way, you can enjoy life to the fullest.

LIFEX CONSTANT 14:   Consider Yourself As Old As You Feel

Our chronological age is simply a certain number of years. What really counts is our functional age.

We all know men and women in their 20s who have middle-aged bodies and who behave and act as if they were 45; and we usually know at least one person in their 70s who can put in a full day's work and still have energy left over for the evening.

This ability to ignore chronological age, and to have the self-image of a person twenty or thirty years younger, is characteristic of many healthful, long-lived persons. For instance, Miss Caroline Algeo of Roseville, California, who observed her 100 birthday a few years ago, said that her recipe for long life had been to ignore her age. A retired teacher, she kept so busy writing that she did not have time to watch the passing years.

"You are only as old as you feel," she said. "And I don't feel old."

Age is an attitude, an awareness, a feeling. When Gary Borkan and Arthur Norris developed their Biological Aging Assessment—an evaluation of twenty-four physical and psychological functions—they found a relationship between the assessment and long life. The more youthful is the assessment of a person's functions, the longer that person lives. Youthfulness, the opposite of aging, can be defined as activity.

Qualities That Make Us Younger

A low functional age will yield vigor, endurance, muscle tone, quick memory, good hearing, swift recovery from illness or setback, a healthy sex life, sound sleep, and a strong zest for life, in addition to other youthful characteristics. The more of these qualities you have, the younger you will look, act, and feel.

Most of these qualities can be acquired or developed. We cannot turn back the clock on our chronological age, but we can easily reverse our functional age by adopting the Lifex Constants.

At least three university studies have each shown that through a program of exercise alone, men and women in their 60s and 70s can lower their physical age between ten and twenty years. For instance, Dr. Herbert DeVries, an exercise physiologist at the University of Southern California, gave a group of men and women aged 52 to 88 a three-hour-a-week exercise program based on both calisthenics and aerobic activity. After only six weeks, many of the participants had regained much of their physical function and vigor and actually reduced their functional age.

How to Reduce Your Functional Age

Central to any desire to reduce functional age, of course, is the need to transform our attitude toward age. To do that, we must consider ourselves only as old as we feel, behave and act.

To ensure that your functional age is below your chronological age, you must observe as many Lifex Constants as possible. Begin with Lifex Constant 5 by exercising regularly and abundantly every day. Then go on to include as many Constants as you can.

Although age is a state of mind largely conditioned by physical and mental activity, also bear in mind that to remain youthful we must stay in touch with contemporary cultural and social values. A number of fit 70-year-olds are physically young but are still back in the 1920s culturally and are out of touch with contemporary social mores.

LIFEX CONSTANT 15:   Develop Sound Sleep Habits

To live long and healthfully, we need a good night's sleep. Observations show that most long-lived people fall asleep quickly and they sleep from six and a half to eight and a half hours, depending on age. The California State Health Department study found that people who sleep seven or eight hours nightly live longest. A study of the profiles of one thousand American centenarians by the Committee for an Extended Lifespan discovered that almost all had retired early and risen early during most of their lives.

If you are one of millions of Americans who spend the night tossing and turning and sleeping fitfully, this indicates that all is not well with your lifestyle habits. Each night, we go through four or five cycles of sleep, each lasting about ninety minutes, and each consisting of four or five stages. Preliminary Stages 1 and 2 are light-to-moderate levels of sleep that last thirty to fifty-five minutes. Our muscles are completely relaxed as we enter deeper Stage 3, which lasts seven to fifteen minutes. Then we pass into Stage 4, the deepest level which may last up to twelve minutes. Finally, we ascend back up into lighter Stage 5 in which we spend most of our time dreaming.

Most somnologists believe that sleep serves two essential purposes. First, deep Stages 3 and 4 are believed essential for physical refreshment and restoration of body cells. Second, dreaming is considered essential for processing newly acquired information and to defuse anxiety and stress by providing answers to upcoming problem situations in our lives.

It Is the Quality of Sleep That Counts

The more time we spend in Stages 3 and 4 and in dreaming, the higher the quality of our sleep. The greater our physical and mental activity during the day, the more time we spend in Stages 3 and 4, and in dreaming, during the night. We experience quality sleep only as we tire our bodies with exercise and as we actively use our minds in creativity, problem-solving or in acquiring new skills and information.

Studies show that our sleep needs diminish as we age. From needing nine hours of sleep at age 12, our sleep needs diminish to only seven hours by age 40, six and a half hours by age 60, and six hours or less by age 80. Many older people continue to spend eight to nine and a half hours in bed when six or seven hours would be biologically more appropriate.

At any age, we get exactly the kind of sleep our lifestyle demands. When we fail to use our minds and bodies, we do not sleep well. If, regardless of our chronological age, we stay active and apply our minds to stimulating and challenging tasks, we continue to enjoy quality sleep.

How to Get a Good Night's Sleep

To sleep soundly for seven or eight hours a night we must create a need for sound sleep. Regarded as essential to sleep are the following Constants:

  Lifex Constant 2. Eliminate All Stimulants
  Lifex Constant 4. Eat Sparingly
  Lifex Constant 5. Exercise Regularly
  Lifex Constant 8. Maintain Recommended Body Weight
  Lifex Constant 23. Keep Growing Intellectually

Constants 11, 12 and 13 are also immensely helpful in minimizing worry and anxiety that can interfere with sleep.

You can also begin to sleep more soundly by rising at the same time every morning, without variation. Go to bed, however, only when tired.

These suggestions offer an infallible springboard to better sleep and use the natural, holistic approach to help you sleep soundly through the night.

10

The Attitudinal Approach
to Life Extension

Gerontologists invariably discover that longevous people have attitudes noticeably different from those of other people. In the United States, this is evident among groups such as the Mormons or the Seventh Day Adventists. In Abkhasia, a citadel of longevity in the Caucasus, researchers have noticed that from early childhood, virtually every youngster grows up fully expecting to live to at least age 90 in vigorous health.

While it may take some inner work to develop the personality traits described in the Lifex Constants in this chapter, the results can be at least as beneficial to your health and longevity as a combination of exercise and low-fat diet.

LIFEX CONSTANT 16: Practice Moderation

A 1980 study at the University of Wisconsin headed by Dr. Robert J. Samp discovered and confirmed many of the Lifex Constants. But the study also revealed that one Constant that occurs without exception in the lives of every longevous person is that of practicing moderation.

Dean Ormish, M.D., and other gerontologists, have concluded that most degenerative diseases are diseases of excess. The are caused because we eat to excess, or use stimulants excessively, or we have a harmful response to stress. People who drive their bodies to excess in training for competitive sports may also stress their bodies so that the joints become inflamed and cartilage is permanently damaged. Training for such events also consumes such excessive amounts of time that it may create time-pressure stress in other areas of life. People who exercise moderately and do nothing to excess may outlive athletes who have been addicted to a single activity.

Even stimulants are less destructive if used in moderation. A number of people who use alcohol very moderately have reached age 100 in relatively good health. A philosophy of practicing moderation in everything we do protects longevous people from the stress of excess.

LIFEX CONSTANT 17:   Develop a Sense of Humor and Cultivate Spontaneity

Laughter and fun stimulate production of endorphins, the body's natural pain-killers. Several studies have demonstrated the therapeutic benefits of playful spontaneity. Dr. O. Carl Simonton found creative play essential in helping patients overcome terminal cancer. Most psychotherapists today consider that laughter and play are among the most effective antidotes to stress.

Becoming a person with a sense of humor is equivalent to transforming ourselves from a Type A or C personality to a Type B. We can accomplish this by deliberately developing the ability to laugh, to play and to welcome spontaneous fun.

Laughing relieves the stress and tension of anger, and anxiety, and increases our energy, efficiency and productivity. The key is to have the capacity to laugh at ourselves and our own mistakes. To do that, we must drop our masks of adult dignity and discard the various roles we play. Doing so frees us to act and look silly. The ability to joke about our fears and to find humor in a discouraging situation indicates that we are in full control of our lives.

So laugh loud and often. Happiness is an attitude we can choose to create.

Revitalize Your Life with Spontaneity

Cultivate your curiosity for new things. Keep an open mind and maintain a youthful enthusiasm for anything new, spontaneous and exciting. Leading a regular, routine life certainly minimizes stress. But every so often we need to break the routine, get out of the rut and have a little unscheduled fun.

LIFEX CONSTANT 18:   Develop a Powerful Will to Live

The intangible life force we call stamina, or the will to live, is another trait shared by many long-lived people. Its existence was confirmed by the Precursor's Study, an ongoing inquiry begun in 1946 based on the psychological profiles of 1,337 medical students at Johns Hopkins University School of Medicine—all of whom eventually became doctors. Results to date show that those doctors with the best health and longevity prognosis all display an unusual strength to withstand disease, fatigue or hardship. They possess a strong resilience to rebound from adversity and an unmistakable harmony between body and mind. Dr. Caroline B. Thomas, professor emeritus at Johns Hopkins University, has defined this combination of factors as "stamina."

Stamina is identical to a strong will to live, which we often call positive thinking. In his book *The Will to Live*, Dr. Arnold Hutschnecker writes: "We die only when we are ready to die. If we truly wish to live, if we have the incentive to live, if we have something to live for, then no matter how sick we may be, no matter how close to death, we do not die. We live because we want to live."

Since Dr. Hutschnecker wrote these words, researchers have confirmed that many people live for as long as they will themselves to attain a goal. People set up deadlines such as living to attend a grandchild's graduation or taking a trip to Europe, or living to be 100. When he studied the lives of 750 people who had recently died, Dr. Phillip R. Kunz of Brigham Young University found that while 46 percent had died in the three months following their birthdays, only 8 percent had died in the three months preceding their birthdays.

Strong Goals Extend Life

The will to live represents all our hopes and aspirations—namely our goals. Goals are our reason for being alive. The mere act of defining a goal means that we intend to live long enough to fulfil it. Our decision to reach a goal affirms that we are in control of our lives and we are playing an active role in fulfilling that goal.

Knowing this, we can create a strong and invincible will to live by setting up a series of clear, strong goals that we can look forward to achieving. Having goals establishes a meaning and purpose for living.

For maximum benefit, our goals should be varied and should include goals for physical activity, mental activity, cultivating positive emotions, and enhancing our career and personal growth. The goals we choose should make maximum use of our talents and abilities. We should also have goals for fun and relaxation, strengthening relationships and family ties, developing love and romance, and widening social contacts.

Consider, for example, having three or more goals to be achieved within six weeks, three or more to be achieved within six months, and three or more to be achieved within six years or longer. Our short-term goals might be to stop smoking within twelve days; to develop a naturally erect carriage within twenty days; and to adapt to the 80-10-10 diet within thirty days. Our intermediate goals might include: to lose twelve pounds within six months; to enroll in the first available class in public speaking; and to spend our fall vacation bicycling through New England. Our long-term goals might be: to live to be 100; to move to a small town within three years; and to own our own business within five years.

Never Be Without Strong Goals

As soon as any goal is achieved, replace it with another. "Without goals, there is no reason to get up in the morning," a spry nonegarian said. "Without goals, our will to live begins to falter." Each goal should state a definite objective and timetable.

It is important to select goals that are clearly attainable. Do not waste time setting impossible goals. Set a goal for something you can definitely reach in a certain period of time.

Observations show that the greater a person's success in life, the longer they may live.

Why Success Makes Us Live Longer

Successful people live longer because they are satisfied and content. Most centenarians feel their lives were well worth living and if they had to do it all over again, they would live their lives the same way. Long-lived people are successful people, even though some may have succeeded in relatively small ways. One way to begin thinking success is to make a list of small successes, each of which you can attain in ten minutes. Achieving a series of small successes will make it easier to achieve larger goals.

Shifting Gears in Your Mind

Creating a powerful will to live is possible for everyone. Through it, we can transform our goals and expectations into inner resources that channel our bodies in the direction we want to go. By developing a powerful will to live, people have overcome the most severe physical limitations.

Everyone has the ability to develop a strong will to live. As Norman Vincent Peale, the originator of positive thinking, wrote: "You can change you life primarily by changing your mental attitude. It's a marvelous fact that nobody needs to remain as he or she is."

Startling Implications of Our Self-Image

Closely intertwined with our goals and will to live is our self-image. Our self-image directs the way we think, believe, act and grow. Our health and longevity are linked to our self-image.

The wonderful thing about our self-image is that if we are not satisfied with it, we can create a new one. Many of us need to improve our sense of self-image. For it is only when we can like and love ourselves that we begin to experience good health. If we are not happy with our self-image, we can create a new blueprint for ourselves.

Remold Your Self-Image

You can create a positive new self-identity by visualizing yourself the way you want to be. Begin to see yourself free of all the things you do not like about yourself, such as being overweight, smoking cigarettes, drinking alcohol, and being selfish. Replace these with positive goals, beliefs, habits and physical factors that reinforce a positive self-image.

Use your existing strengths, potentials and talents as building blocks. Congratulate yourself for having these good points and forgive yourself for your weaknesses. Build the framework of your new self-image around your existing strengths.

The goals upon which your new self-image is based are often similar to the goals which comprise your will to live. In fact, your will to live is probably an integral part of your overall self-image. The more you are able to accept your new self-image, the greater will be your self-esteem and self-worth. As your attitude becomes increasingly positive, you will reduce susceptibility to accidents and to stress-related disease.

Almost immediately, you will begin to live out your new image of yourself. You will begin to feel like a worthwhile person. You will feel confident and secure.

LIFEX CONSTANT 19:   Cultivate a Loving, Friendly Attitude

Being a loving person does not imply that you must behave like a saint. There are gruff, outwardly brusque people who have a heart of gold within. People express love in different ways. It is important, though, to distinguish between being a loving, caring, nurturing Type-B person and being a Type C person who lives to serve and please others. To become a loving Type-B person you may be quite assertive in saying No to anything that might pressure you. You cannot afford to let yourself be used by others. You can feel free to turn down unwanted responsibility and still be a loving person.

Making Your Feelings Transparent

To love is equivalent to accepting other people without being critical or judgmental. Another characteristic of loving people is their willingness to reveal their deepest feelings. To do this, we must first drop the mask of pretentiousness and artificiality that separates us from others. By opening ourselves completely and hiding nothing—by becoming emotionally transparent—we will immediately find ourselves becoming closer to other people. Revealing our deepest feelings, and telling the truth about ourselves, makes us emotionally vulnerable to feeling hurt. But that is a risk we must take if we are to become trusting and warm toward others.

A University of Michigan study recently demonstrated that it is much healthier to present our real, honest, sensitive self to the world rather than to suppress our negative emotions. The study showed that people who are unable to express their emotions (typical Type C's) suffer from a wide range of degenerative diseases. In contrast, people who express their emotions freely seldom suffer from degenerative diseases. Such people do not find it necessary to keep a distance between themselves and others.

Being a loving person means being completely open and honest. It means being free of resentment or desire to retaliate. Loving people do not take their anger out on others. They are generous and assist those in need whenever possible. (It does not mean that we must automatically loan money to bail out financially irresponsible friends and relatives. There are frequently more deserving causes to which we can make a contribution. As you become a really loving person, you will discover that it is impossible to please everyone or to expect that everyone is going to like you.) As you develop an unselfish love of yourself and others, the healthier you will become and the longer you are likely to live.

11

The Sociological Approach to Life Extension

All around the world, longevous people are proving that it is never too late to fall in love, marry, or even to have children. Our need for companionship, affection, human contact and sex persist to the very end of life. The following Lifex Constants demonstrate that if these needs are not met, life may be shortened. To maximize our longevity potential, we need an abundance of successful relationships, including a compatible and stable marriage with accompanying family life.

LIFEX CONSTANT 20: Develop a Supportive Network of Friends and Relatives

A number of studies have proved that close relationships are an essential part of living longer and have a salutary effect on health. An unusual study was made of the inhabitants of Roseto, Pennsylvania, a town settled almost entirely by Italians and rich in Italian tradition and culture. For years, observers had noted the almost total absence of heart disease among Roseto's residents. During the 1950s and 1960s, researchers in droves descended on Roseto to measure blood pressure and cholesterol levels and to investigate the diet and exercise patterns of its inhabitants. Finally, after several years of intense investigation, a computer analysis came up with an answer.

Neither diet nor exercise were responsible for Roseto's low cardiac-mortality and longer life-expectancy. The intimacy, love and support provided by the town's close-knit multi-generation Italian families was responsible for extending the lives of the inhabitants.

Friends Help Us Live Longer

Humans survive best in the presence of close, loving, relationships. This was demonstrated by studies of married Protestant clergy whom, it was found, invariably outlive celibate Catholic priests. Other studies show that people are nourished by friendship and the support friends provide. One study by Dr. Lisa Berkman of the California Department of Public Health reported that people with few social contacts are two and a half to three times more likely to die prematurely than people with more active social lives. The study showed that people with few family contacts or friends, or with few social contacts through groups and organizations, were in a high-risk category. The same study reported that the death rate for widows exposed to any form of stress is three to thirteen times greater than for married women.

Although it is believed that loneliness suppresses the immune system, the exact mechanism which contributes to death among the lonely has not been clearly identified. We do know that we are as healthy and long-lived as our relationships make us. Strong social bonds and ties, together with hugging, touching, loving and affection, are as essential to wellness as are exercise and balanced eating.

Profiles of healthy centenarians show that the vast majority value close relationships. They seek and foster close relationships throughout their lives. They are invariably supportive and ready to help others. If a spouse dies, the survivor remarries if possible. Most centenarians have had several children and most have enjoyed the support of extensive multi-generation families. Even those who experience a bad marriage seldom withdraw into solitary activities. They always seem ready to take the risk and marry again.

Parenthood Extends Life

Records show that women who have three or four children outlive childless women or women who have only one child. However, mortality rates gradually rise for women with seven or more children. Having children releases a surge of estrogen during pregnancy and nursing that may furnish a considerable degree of protection against breast cancer throughout life.

Childless couples frequently see themselves as failures and may experience emotional disorders. By contrast, married men or women who come home from a hard day at work to find a loving, supportive family waiting, experience minimum damage from job stress and they quickly recover.

Unfortunately, today's nuclear family is often scattered and the generations seldom see each other. In many contemporary families, each member is often so busy and concerned with individual activities that the benefits of family cohesiveness are being lost.

Health Benefits in Large Families

Undoubtedly, people are healthier and live longer when part of a traditional, multi-generation family. Such families still exist, particularly among Mormons and Seventh Day Adventists.

The fact that many centenarians have spent their entire lives close to their birthplace has enabled them to enjoy the support and continued involvement of a multi-generation family. Close family-ties with several generations assure older family members of a support system. A loving family provides such essential ingredients for long life as a sense of warmth and a feeling of being needed and wanted. The love and acceptance of each member's imperfections creates the type of personality that is flexible and able to swiftly adjust to change. This same support, love and acceptance allows family members to be themselves and to express themselves freely.

Statistics show that people in compatible and permanent marriages, with accompanying family life, outlive single people by an appreciable margin. Figures released by the Health Insurance Institute show that divorced men run twice the risk of heart disease or cancer and seven times the risk of cirrhosis as do married men. When a spouse dies, the surviving partner runs an increased risk of dying within the following six months.

Living Alone Is Hazardous to Your Health
Much of the evidence showing that married people are more resistant to disease originated with the Midtown Manhattan Study made during the 1950s. This and similar studies made in the United States, showed that men who were separated or divorced and living alone lost eight years from their life expectancy. Widowers living alone lost seven years; however, widowed, separated or divorced men who were not living alone but who were sharing a household with friends or family, lost only half as many years from their life expectancy.

For women, loss of love proved less disastrous. Separated or divorced women living alone lost only four years from their life expectancy while widowed women living alone gave up only three and a half years. Divorced or widowed women who remained heads of families lost only two years of life.

For men and women who have never been married, deprivation of love is less severe. Men who have never married but live alone lose two years of life expectancy for each unmarried decade after age 25 while women lose only one year.

In all cases, the studies found that loss of love shortens life. But findings also demonstrated that single men and women who lived with friends or family lost only half as many years of life expectancy as single people who lived alone. It was also discovered that single people who were active in a number of social and community organizations and who enjoyed a wide circle of friends experienced scarcely any loss in life expectancy at all.

Some of these statistics, gathered several decades ago when a definite social stigma was attached to being unmarried, are being questioned today.

We now have a new breed of singles who are single by choice. While no significant studies have been done, indications are that depression among modern singles is little higher than among married people (many more of whom are now childless than was the case several decades ago).

A study by Kaud J. Helsing of Johns Hopkins Training Center for Public Health, released in 1981, showed a marked decrease in deaths of surviving spouses compared to figures obtained during the 1950s and earlier. One explanation is that most earlier deaths were due to infections resulting from suppression of the immune system, and antibiotics available today have overcome many diseases.

How can we best cultivate the kind of close relationships that seem to extend life? First, by creating a compatible and permanently stable marriage that includes an accompanying family life; and second, by cultivating as many friends as possible and by being active in as many social organizations and groups as we can.

Proof of the health benefits accruing from contacts other than through family life appeared in the Surgeon General's 1979 report on *Health Promotion and Disease Prevention*. The report found extensive evidence of the beneficial role of belonging to neighborhood institutions such as churches, ethnic and social clubs, fraternal and community organizations, and similar local networks. Belonging to these organizations helps people gain control over their lives, reduces feelings of alienation, and improves ability to deal with life's stresses and problems.

Secrets of Successful Relationships

The main qualities of a successful marriage are: a willingness to put the needs and well-being of the other person ahead of your own; total acceptance of each other without trying to change the other person; spending time with each other; honest, open communication; a willingness to make a determined effort to create a happy relationship; a recognition by the husband that women are totally equal in every way; and recognition by the wife that men may have difficulty in expressing their deepest feelings.

Studies by Lak Bulusu, a British government statistician, found that a wide age gap between marriage partners can create stress that shortens life. English records show that women in their 50s or 60s who are ten to fifteen years older than their husbands have a mortality rate significantly higher than normal. Women 55 to 64 married to much younger men had a death rate almost double that of women married to men of roughly equal years. In contrast, men married to younger women experienced no increased health risk until the age gap exceeded fifteen years. Men married to women fifteen or more years their junior begin to show signs of increased stress.

According to a Duke University study, the happiest marriages for mature people are those in which the wife is several years younger than the husband; the husband is at least as intelligent and well-educated as the wife; and there is frequent sexual activity.

Contrasting sociological levels between marriage partners can threaten the health of the male. Data collected by the Human Population Laboratory in Berkeley, California, reveal that marriages in which a highly educated husband has a low-status, low-paid job (such as a Ph.D., working as a sales clerk) while a wife who never completed college has worked her way up to become head of a department at a high salary, threatens both the ego and the life expectancy of the husband. Men in such situations have a heart disease risk eleven times that of the average married man. The same data shows that marriages succeed best when both husband and wife are from the same socio-economic and cultural backgrounds.

Social Bonds Are Essential

When a follow-up study was done on the California State Health Department's investigation of the effects of social and community ties on longevity, in every age group examined, those men and women with the most numerous social contacts had the lowest mortality rate. Conversely, those with fewest contacts had the highest death rate.

Based on study results, researchers offered this advice. Surround yourself with friends and family who can support you and whom you can support. Everyone, for example, should have at least two close confidants. Try to stay married if you can and develop a close, stable relationship with your spouse. If you cannot, then live with a friend or relative.

If you live alone, consider offering to share your home with a friend or someone else who could help relieve loneliness. Invite new acquaintances to your home. Be receptive and reach out.

How to Banish Loneliness

Loneliness is a major threat to health and long life, but loneliness can be swiftly overcome. To do so, we should carefully avoid setting ourselves apart from others. We should avoid judging people and categorizing them by race, religion, recreation or occupation. We should also avoid accentuating differences that we believe may win approval for us, but which set us apart and isolate us from others. Instead of emphasizing differences, look for things you have in common with others.

A successful relationship also requires an investment of time. Be prepared to spend some time with your spouse and family or with friends. And most importantly, friendships occur only when you make a contribution. You might consider becoming active in working for a volunteer or conservation group or a political organization. Through helping others you help expand your own contacts. The greater your contribution, the more friends you will make.

If loneliness is a problem, organize an immediate campaign to end it. Put your time and effort into seeking out ways to meet people. Join church, social, hobby and recreational clubs. Get out of the house and begin to meet and interact with people. At all costs, avoid isolating yourself. As you meet others, try to include people of all ages as your friends—especially younger people through whom you can stay in touch with new developments and new uses of language.

Do not be intimidated if you are middle-aged or older. America's mushrooming older population has spawned hundreds of senior dating services and senior singles groups galore. In large retirement communities, singles bars flourish and community newspapers are filled with classified ads from retirees seeking dates. If you are a woman of mature years, do not be shy about contacting a potential marriage mate. Older single men, grown unaccustomed to dating, often become shy and lack confidence. Many actually welcome a woman who takes the initiative.

You may also find that through adopting the Lifex Constants you no longer have as much in common with your former friends. In this case, consider contacting health-oriented groups such as a local chapter of the American Natural Hygiene Society. Through joining organizations, you can make new friends.

LIFEX CONSTANT 21:   Enjoy Regular Sexual Activity

Regular sexual activity with one permanent partner is a Constant found among almost all married centenarians and long-lived people. Statistics reveal that the stimulation, intimacy, and relaxation associated with lovemaking adds an average of two years to life expectancy.

The National Institutes on Aging report that most people are able to enjoy sexual activity throughout life. A Duke University study of 255 men aged 60 to 94 found that half those in their 60s still engaged in sexual activity while 15 percent were still active in their 80s. More surprisingly, 10 percent of the men studied reported an increase in sexual activity as they grew older. The study concluded that most men and women can continue to enjoy sex until age 80 or later. Researchers also observed that those who were most sexually satisfied in their younger years, and who maintained a positive attitude about sex, were those who enjoyed sex most in the later years.

We Do Not Have to Be Sexually Inactive at Sixty-Five

While a slow, gradual decline in output of sperm and testosterone begins in males after age 40, and a gradual cessation of function in the ovaries of females occurs with menopause, sex drive persists unabated in both men and women until very late in life. So it is hardly surprising that after reaching 40, many couples find that their sex drive is stronger than before.

These findings disprove the widely-held belief that sexual desire and performance diminish almost totally by age 65, or that the physical exertion of lovemaking may bring on a heart attack in older people. Many women, as well as some men, give up lovemaking after age 50 for no other reason than that they subscribe to these myths.

In reality, sexual activity is a functional component of a long, happy life. Fit, healthy older men and women continue to derive as much pleasure from lovemaking as do younger people. The only difference is that older men take slightly longer to achieve an erection and to reach a climax. The amount of ejaculated sperm also decreases. The result is that an older man is able to maintain an erection longer before climaxing than most younger men—an effect which heightens satisfaction for both partners.

Although most women cease to produce estrogen and progesterone with the end of the menstrual cycle at around age 45, this has no effect on sexual libido or enjoyment. Many women, in fact, report enjoying sex more after menopause when anxiety about pregnancy disappears.

The principal barrier to sex in the later years is finding an active and interesting partner. The fact is that millions of older people lack sexual vigor. Their loss of vigor is almost invariably associated with an unhealthy lifestyle built around such habits as indulgence in alcohol or cigarettes; or in high-fat diet that leads to overweight and lack of exercise and, eventually, to diabetes.

A number of common prescription and over-the-counter medications may also adversely affect sex drive and performance. Anti-hypertensive medications, anti-depressants, tranquilizers, peptic ulcer drugs, barbiturates and other sleeping pills, painkillers, and anti-cholinergenics (eye medication) may all subdue sexual desire. Unresolved stress arising from worry, fear and anxiety can also create impotence.

12

The Actualization Approach
to Life Extension

Self-actualization is the term used by humanist psychologist Abraham Maslow to describe people who maximize their potential in every area of life. To actualize your life means making the most of it in every way. It means continuing to grow throughout life and attaining success through working at an occupation that challenges you. It means experiencing pride and achievement through doing the very best work that you can. It means using your mind and memory to constantly explore new ideas, to solve problems and to make choices.

The more we actualize ourselves, the better our health and the longer we live. The annals are filled with examples of self-actualized people who made major contributions to entertainment and the arts and sciences late in life. Eubie Blake, a jazz pianist, made a comeback in his 80s and played till age 100. In 1982, Ruth Hutchinson, the world's oldest rock-and-roll disc jockey, was still going strong at age 88. Cellist Pablo Casals played until his death at 96. In 1983, Dorothy Fuldheim, America's oldest newswomen, was still broadcasting regularly at age 89. In 1942 at age 73, Myrtle Youngberg of Harper, Kansas became a judge and spent the next fourteen years hearing juvenile and probate cases. Through observing most of the Lifex Constants, Myrtle Youngberg went on to become a centenarian. When asked for advice on her hundredth birthday in 1979, she said, "Believe in what you want and go all out for it. Believe in yourself and you can do anything."

LIFEX CONSTANT 22:   Work at Something Meaningful and Challenging Throughout Life

Some years ago, the National Institutes of Health made an eleven-year investigation of six hundred possible variables that contribute to longevity.

They found that the most significant factor in extending life is not exercise, diet, heredity or taking nutritional supplements, but the degree of satisfaction we derive from our work.

Another study made in 1982 by Duke University Center for the Study of Aging found that the best indicator of long life for men over 60 is their satisfaction with work. Without exception, study after study has correlated the ability to continue to work at a meaningful, creative, and useful job with living longer.

By comparison, compulsory retirement has been identified as the leading sub-clinical cause of death for men. A study by Dr. Ward Cassells of Beth Israel Hospital, Boston, found that retired men had a risk of heart disease 80 percent greater than men still working. Being forced to stop work at an arbitrary retirement age can be a stressful and traumatic event that leads to dramatic lifestyle changes. People who identify themselves closely with their work frequently link their self-image with their occupation. Retirement destroys their self-image. Those who lack the flexibility to adapt to these difficult adjustments often find retirement intolerable.

Destructive Effects of Compulsory Retirement

In almost all primitive and agricultural societies, the elderly enjoy dignity and respect. They continue to work at healthful occupations throughout life and the work keeps them fit and mentally alert. In modern industrialized societies, many people destroy their health through dehumanizing work. At 65 or earlier, most American workers are given a gold watch and forced into retirement.

The A.M.A. Committee on Aging considers arbitrary retirement and denial of work opportunity a serious threat to health. Several studies have proved that the longer people work past 60, the healthier they are and the longer they live. All available evidence suggests that unless they can continue to contribute to the lives of others, life expectancy is shortened for people who retire. Only by contributing and working can a person achieve full status as a member of society.

The Life-Extending Power of Satisfying Work

It is not so much our need to work that motivates longevity as our need to contribute and make a difference through leading a useful and purposeful life. Millions of Americans who hold stressful jobs have retired and launched more satisfying second careers.

If we have a satisfying and enjoyable occupation already, we will live longer by continuing to work at it for as long as possible. If our work appears boring, monotonous, stressful and unrewarding, we will stay healthier by either retiring or making a mid-life career change to a more meaningful occupation.

Thus, working at any kind of occupation does not necessarily extend life. People live longest only when they can continue to work at an occupation that is enjoyable and satisfying. Gerontologists have defined a satisfying occupation as one that has all or most of these qualities: You should either be your own boss or be free to make most of your own decisions; you should not be under close supervision. The occupation should make maximum use of your skills and talents; it should call for innovation and creativity; and it should encourage you to reach out for high achievement. It should allow you to do the very best work that you can. It should allow you to rise through promotion, or to succeed in reaching a position of eminence in your chosen field. You should be able to work at your own pace free of deadlines or pressures. You should be under no compulsion to retire and you should be able to work for as long as you wish. The work should be useful and should contribute to the lives of others. Doing it should make you feel good about yourself.

High-Achievement Occupations

Among occupations that generally fit these requirements are: self-employed persons and sole proprietors of businesses; medical specialists; top corporate executives; artists, authors, playwrights, composers and craftsmen; orchestra conductors and musicians; actors; airline pilots; foresters; organic farmers and gardeners; protestant ministers; educators; scientists; non-mechanized mail carriers; attorneys; members of Congress or the United States Senate; top ranking military officers; and Justices of the United States Supreme Court. People in these occupations tend to outlive the general public. Obviously, most of these are high-achievement occupations.

Strenuous outdoor work is also a powerful stimulator of long life, provided the worker has total autonomy and works in a pollution-free environment as do organic gardeners, farmers and most foresters.

While it may appear that most of these occupations are out of reach, literally millions of Americans with modest talents have become self-employed and they operate a small business.

Life-Shortening Occupations

A variety of studies have shown that people who hold tightly supervised, lower echelon jobs have a life expectancy well below average. Job-stress specialists, such as Professor Robert Karasek of New York's Columbia University, explain that jobs like these often involve repetitive, mind-dulling work in an authoritarian, tightly supervised environment. Assembly-line workers must frequently keep pace with machines or electronic devices. When these are speeded up, the worker's stress is intensified.

Adding to stress is the fact that today's workers are more highly educated and have higher expectations for a meaningful and satisfying career. But, their skills and talents are often underutilized—an experience that leads to chronic frustration. Professor Karasek reportedly estimates that 25 percent of all Americans have stress-related work problems that could lead to heart disease or similar degenerative disease.

Other jobs can shorten life because of the stress of working under pressure to meet tight deadlines and schedules. A list of life-shortening occupations would include: newsmen, journalists and correspondents; employees in mines and factories; cooks and waitresses; garment workers; telephone operators; cashiers; middle-management executives; workers in public relations and advertising; dental and lab technicians; bank tellers; policemen, firemen, mechanics, laborers, secretaries and workers who use video display terminals.

These jobs can be highly stressful because they often involve boring, monotonous work under close supervision, which allows minimum opportunity for independent decision-making. For example, being a semi-skilled employee can cut six months from life expectancy while being a laborer, waitress or assembly-line worker can reduce life expectancy by two to four years.

Thus, stressful work can be as destructive to health as smoking a pack of cigarettes per day. British studies have also revealed that men in stressful occupations bring their stress home with them so that their wives, too, tend to suffer from stress.

New and Exciting Options to Actualize Our Lives

Options for maximizing our life and health within the framework of modern society include finding an occupation you enjoy. If you already have a satisfying and enjoyable occupation, continue to work at it for as long as possible. Choose work that is interesting and challenges your creativity. The more stimulating and creative your work, the more it fortifies you against life's stresses.

If your work is stressful, purposeless and unsatisfying, or if it involves stressful commuting, consider making a career change. Make a list of occupational goals you would like to achieve and begin looking at alternatives. Most centenarians made several career changes to meet changing economic conditions during their long lives. A number of longevous men found new occupations every ten or fifteen years. Consider going into business for yourself. Literally hundreds of overstressed middle-management executives have resigned their high-paid careers and found greater satisfaction through making a change.

Until you can change occupations, use Lifex Constants 11, 12 and 13 to help take the stress out of your present job. You can also compensate for job stress by taking up an enjoyable hobby in which you can excel, by making your own decisions, and by working at your own pace.

Another alternative may be voluntary retirement. Surveys show that many people who formerly worked at stressful jobs derive pleasure from the lack of regimentation and from the autonomy of retirement living. But most soon tire of fishing and playing golf and seek out something else to do. The majority feel a need to contribute through part-time or volunteer work.

If retirement is forced on you, respond in a healthy way by planning for a second career.

Alternatively, you can continue to contribute through staying busy in volunteer work or community affairs. In any case, do not settle for menial work. Become productively involved in the kind of work you do best. Take on new challenges; grow and move ahead toward higher achievements.

If you can, contribute through hobbies or recreations. When Dr. Clifford Graves of La Jolla, California, retired from medical practice, he and his wife devoted themselves full-time to organizing and operating non-profit bicycle tours for adults throughout the world.

The late Scott Nearing and his wife Helen, who pioneered the self-sufficient homestead movement, inspired thousands of Americans to forsake the supermarket and the job market and to find greater satisfaction through living off the land. By living in harmony with nature, and following a lifestyle which included almost all the Lifex Constants, Scott Nearing actively contributed to the lives of others until the final day of his life at age 100.

A 1980 study of aging in America by the American Health Foundation reported that Americans over 65 who perform volunteer work experienced better health than those who did not work. Active participation and involvement in helping others offers great personal fulfillment. Any form of social activism is important to optimal functioning throughout life.

LIFEX CONSTANT 23:   Keep Growing Intellectually

Observations show that most longevous people have above-average intelligence and remain mentally healthy and mentally active throughout life. One twelve-year study by the National Institutes of Health found that people who live longest tended to have a higher I.Q., to be more emotionally stable, and to have a better adjusted personality than the general public. Professional people outlive the general public by three to five years. Longitudinal studies by such organizations as the Metropolitan Life Insurance Company and AT&T reveal that, in modern times, intelligent and well-educated people have a life expectancy at least two years greater than average.

By contrast, people with fewer than eight years of schooling have a mortality rate that is two and a half years shorter than normal.

While records show that more than half of all longevous people have received higher education, there remains a large unexplained number of centenarians who had little education. Some were actually illiterate. However, despite lack of opportunity for higher education, almost all these long-lived people had above-average intelligence.

The key is the ability to acquire wisdom and understanding as a result of intelligence and education. Another goal is to remain mentally active throughout life.

You Do Not Need a Ph.D., to Live Long and Healthfully

Gerontologists themselves have been unable to establish a direct causal relationship between higher education and longevity. Higher education opens up a wide spectrum of such socio-economic advantages as higher income; high-status occupations with greater autonomy and less stress; better medical care; better living conditions with less crowding, noise and stress; and fewer occupational risk hazards. Thus, it is difficult to isolate higher education as a direct cause of long life.

Educated people are also more likely to read the latest health advice and to have a greater awareness of the need for exercise, a low-fat diet and stress-management. Uneducated people, by contrast, may be discouraged by peer pressure from adopting healthful habits. It is difficult to break away from friends whose lives may be centered around life-threatening habits.

Nonetheless, many intelligent people in lower socio-economic brackets have had the wisdom to transform their habits. On the other hand, an appreciable percentage of people with higher education still lack the wisdom to follow healthful lifestyles.

Sifting below the surface of these trends and studies, we find that intelligence and wisdom are basic keys to long life. Coupled with this is the fact that intelligent people at all socio-economic levels tend to use their minds actively and constantly.

To live long and healthfully does not require a high I.Q. All we need is the intelligence to recognize the wisdom of adopting a healthy lifestyle.

Ways to Stimulate Your Creativity and Imagination

Reading is an excellent mental exercise because it forces the mind to create images and it stimulates thoughts and ideas. Listening to tapes also stimulates imagery.

We can exercise the mind in dozens of other pleasant ways. Try writing letters instead of telephoning. Visit art galleries and museums. Play mind-taxing games like chess, bridge, word games, or computer games. Puzzles of all types are stimulating, from crossword and jig-saw puzzles to books of puzzles and mind-teasers.

Think about getting a home computer and teaching yourself to use it. Discuss news items with others. Keep active at hobbies and consider taking up new ones.

While no proof exists that returning to school and acquiring higher education later in life enhances life expectancy, the mere desire for learning is a desire for increased mental activity. Opportunities for adult education are endless. Just about every state university and college offers free or inexpensive college-level courses or vocational training to adults of all ages. Many institutions have extensive continuing-education programs. Attending classes not only stimulates the mind but provides new contacts and social interaction.

Never overlook opportunities to teach yourself. Think about making science a hobby. Consider taking up astronomy, cosmology, or botany or biology. Every kind of creative activity sharpens the mind and that helps extend life.

LIFEX CONSTANT 24: Seek Maximum Independence

People who enjoy a high degree of independence and autonomy in making choices—in both job and family life—tend to have a high wellness-profile. These are people who have taken control of their lives and who experience minimum stress.

People listed in *Who's Who* have a life expectancy 19 percent greater than the general population. Although higher education and greater affluence undoubtedly play a role, a strong factor is believed to be the greater autonomy available to people who reach positions of eminence. Many prominent people in *Who's Who* frequently exercise control over their own lives and achieve greater satisfaction with less stress. They control their own destinies and set their own pace. When Dr. Joseph T. Freedman, former president of the Gerontological Society, studied the lives of 14,622 men throughout history, he found that the longest-lived were those who held positions of greatest responsibility.

This phenomenon is not limited to top echelon people but exists at all levels of society. A National Research Council study of ten thousand men drafted into the Army in 1944 found that the higher their rank at discharge, the longer they lived. The mortality rate for privates was twice that for sergeants. A British study also reported that blue-collar workers aged 35 had the same heart disease risk as executives aged 47. The blue-collar workers indulged twice as heavily in cigarettes and alcohol as did the executives. Twice as many were overweight.

Take Control of Your Own Destiny

Gerontologists explain that at any social level, the greater our autonomy, the longer we live. The reason, they believe, is that people who are in control of a situation experience much less stress than those who feel they have no control. People in control are able to escape from a stressful situation and are then able to quickly recover. When we can control the source of our stress, the situation is much less damaging. Self-employed people suffer less from stress because they can turn it off at any time. By contrast, a worker on a speeded-up assembly line has no control over the source of his stress.

To take control of your own destiny means to take charge of every aspect in your life that you can control. Then accept what you cannot control and stop worrying about it.

LIFEX CONSTANT 25:   Be Ready to Take Prudent Risks

We begin to feel old when we stop growing, and we stop growing when we become unwilling to take prudent risks. To risk is to learn and grow, to be open to change, and to be mildly adventuresome.

Risks That Extend Life

Only by taking an occasional prudent risk, or by trying something new, can we add zest to our lives and life to our years. Taking an occasional chance equips us to deal with worry and fear. Naturally, you should not risk your savings on a wildly speculative venture. But you might risk a date or a ride on a roller coaster or on something else you have never done before. If your job is unsatisfying, you could take a chance on changing careers. You could take up a new recreation or a new activity you have never tried before.

Long-lived people are not afraid to experiment with new ideas. Thousands have extended their lives through taking up new ideas for healthful living, such as a low-fat diet or exercise, long before these things were proven beneficial by science.

Only through taking an occasional prudent risk can we ever succeed. Observations show that many healthy centenarians are adventuresome people who are willing to take calculated risks to succeed. However, they are also careful to avoid unnecessary risks.

LIFEX CONSTANT 26:   Have Faith in Something Spiritual

Believing in and relying on something spiritual is an effective and powerful stress-management technique. A study of the profiles of one thousand American centenarians by the Committee for an Extended Lifespan found that almost every centenarian had strong religious faith, and that they relied on that power to guide them toward the best possible solution. Meanwhile, secure in their faith, they were able to relax and enjoy life.

Although many centenarians do not follow a formal religion, many believe in a power greater than themselves. They believe that life is essentially good. They try to see the best in everything and everybody and to overlook life's imperfections. Such an attitude creates strong feelings of security and warmth and lessens any feelings of being alone.

As a result, spiritual faith has been found to be the most effective and dependable way of transforming stress into non-stress.

Numerous studies on the Mormons, Seventh Day Adventists and other religious groups indicate a strong correlation between religious beliefs and improved health and longevity. One advantage of group worship is that it increases the bonds of human contact with a strong and loving support system.

Religion focuses on the positive aspects of life and people. Observations suggest that thinking positive thoughts, and seeing the world as a friendly place, releases beneficial hormones that stimulate health. If, by contrast, we view the world as threatening and see life as a series of problems and difficulties, we turn on the Fight or Flight response. The body is then constantly exposed to hostile feelings of anger and fear that can trigger illness.

Through any form of meditation that focuses our awareness on positive qualities, we feel a powerful force is working for us. By turning over our problems to a higher power for solution and guidance, we experience a tremendous release of tension.

Our search for spiritual faith has created an enormous variety of religions and types of worship. Among those with a definite holistic slant toward health and longevity are the Seventh Day Adventist, Mormon, Unity, and Christian Science churches as well as a number of oriental philosophies including hatha yoga.

LIFEX CONSTANT 27:   Make Clear, Bold, and Unequivocal Choices

To choose wisely, we must distinguish between making decisions and making choices. To make a decision, list all the pros and cons, weigh them and then decide how to act.

Much of the time, we are not aware of the pros and cons involved; we must make a choice, not a decision. Through making a free choice, we have control over, and are responsible for, our decision.

To make bold, clear-cut choices means being in full charge of our lives. Healthful, long-lived people do not live in fear of being unable to choose. Unless it becomes obvious that they have made a mistake, once they have made a choice, they stick with it.

The choice, therefore, is ours. All we need to know in order to live a long and healthful life is within these pages. The rest is strictly up to us.

Bibliography

Books

Aero, Rita. *The Complete Book of Longevity.* G.P. Putnam, 1980.

Alexander, F. Mathias. *The Resurrection of the Body.* Delta Books, 1974.

Ardell, Donald, Ph.D. *Fourteen Days to a Wellness Lifestyle.* Whatever Publishing Inc., 1982.

_____ *High Level Wellness.* Rodale-Bantam Books, 1977.

Ballantine, Rudoph, M.D. *Diet and Nutrition: a Holistic Approach.* Honesdale, Pennsylvania; Himalayan Institute, 1978.

Barker, Sarah. *The Alexander Technique.* Bantam Books, 1978.

Baron, Howard C., M.D. *Varicose Veins.* William Morrow, 1979,

Bennet, William, M.D.; Gurin, Joel. *The Dieter's Dilemma: Eating Less and Weighing More.* Basic Books, 1982.

Benson, Herbert, M.D. *The Mind-Body Effect.* Simon and Schuster, 1979.

Blanding, Forrest. *The Pulse Point Program.* Random House, 1982.

Bruhn, John G., M.D.; Wolf, Stewart. *The Roseto Story: An Anatomy of Health.* University of Oklahoma Press, 1979.

Bresler, David, M.D. *Free Yourself from Pain.* Simon and Schuster, 1979.

Burns, David D., M.D. *Feeling Good.* William Morrow, 1980.

Butler, Robert N. *Why Survive? Being Old in America.* Harper and Row, 1975.

Carlson, Rick J. *The End of Medicine.* John Wiley and Sons, 1975.

Casewit, Curtis. *Quit Smoking.* Para Research, 1983.

_____ *The Stop Smoking Book For Teens.* Julian Messner, 1980.

Chandra, R. K., M.D. *Nutrition, Immunity and Infection.* Plenum Press, 1982.

Clark, Linda. *Rejuvenation.* Devin-Adair, 1978.

Crapo, Lawrence, M.D.; Fries, James, M.D. *Vitality and Aging.* W. H. Freeman, 1981.

Cousins, Norman. *Anatomy of an Illness*, W. W. Norton, 1979.

_____ *Human Options*. W. W. Norton, 1982.

_____ *The Healing Heart*. W. W. Norton, 1983.

Cutler, Richard. *Aging, Carcinogenesis and Radiation Biology*. Plenum Press, 1976.

De Beauvoir, Simone. *The Coming of Age*. G. P. Putnam, 1972.

DeVries, Herbert A., Ph.D.; Dianne Hales. *Fitness After Fifty*. Scribner's, 1982.

Dickinson, Peter. *The Fires of Autumn*. Drake Publishers, 1974.

Dudley, Ronald, M.D. *How to Survive Being Alive*. New American Library, 1979.

Eyton, Audrey. *The F-Plan Diet*. Crown Publishers, 1983.

Farquhar, John W., M.D. *The American Way of Life Need Not Be Hazardous to Your Health*. Stanford, California; Stanford Alumni Association, 1978.

Feldenkrais, Moshe. *Awareness Through Movement*. Harper and Row, 1972.

Ferguson, Marilyn. *The Aquarian Conspiracy*. J. P. Tarcher, 1980.

Ford, Norman D. *Good Health Without Drugs*. St. Martins Press, 1978.

_____ *Secrets of Staying Young and Living Longer*. Harian, 1979.

_____ *Natural Ways to Relieve Pain*. Harian, 1980.

_____ *Arthritis*. Prentice Hall, 1981.

_____ *Mind-ing Your Body*. Autumn Press, 1982.

_____ *Good Night*. Para Research, 1983.

Friedman, Meyer, M.D.; Rosenman, Ray H., M.D. *Type A Behaviour and Your Heart*. Fawcett, 1978.

_____ *The Heart: Update V.* McGraw-Hill, 1981.

Freudenberger, Herbert J.; Richardson, Geraldine. *Burnout—The High Cost of Success*. Doubleday, 1980.

Fry, William, M.D.; Allen, Melanie. *Make 'em Laugh*. Science and Behavior, 1976.

Galton, Lawrence, M.D. *How Long Will I Live?* McMillan, 1976.

Georgakas, Dan. *The Methuselah Factors*. Simon and Schuster, 1980.

Gillies, Jerry. *Psychological Immortality; Using Your Mind to Extend Your Life*. Richard Marek, 1981.

Hafen, Brent, Q., Ph.D. *Medical Self-Care and Assessment*. Morton Publishing, 1983.

Harris, Raymond, M.D. *Guide to Fitness After Fifty*. Plenum Press, 1977.

Hoffer, Abram, Ph.D., M.D. *Orthomolecular Nutrition*. Keats Publishing, 1978.

Jaffe, Dennis T., M.D. *Healing From Within*. Knopf, 1980.

Kendig, Frank; Hutton, Richard. *Lifespans*. Holt, Rhinehart and Winston, 1979.

Kent, Saul. *The Life Extension Revolution.* William Morrow, 1980.

Kugler, Hans J., Ph.D. *Slowing Down the Aging Process.* Harcourt, Brace, 1973.

Langone, John. *Long Life.* Little, Brown; 1978.

_____ *What We Know and Are Learning About the Aging Process.* Little, Brown; 1978.

Lamb, Lawrence E., M.D. *Get Ready for Immortality.* Harper and Row, 1974.

Leaf, Alexander, M.D. *Youth in Old Age.* McGraw Hill, 1975.

Levinson, Daniel, Ph.D. *Seasons of a Man's Life.* Ballantine Books, 1978.

Lesser, Michael, M.D. *Nutrition and Vitamin Therapy.* Bantam Books, 1981.

Litvak, Stuart, Ph.D. *Unstress Yourself.* Ross-Erikson, 1980.

Luce, Gay Gaer. *Your Second Life.* Delacorte, 1979.

Lynch, James J., Ph.D. *The Broken Heart; the Medical Consequences of Loneliness.* Basic Books, 1977.

Mann, John A. *Secrets of Life Extension.* Harbor Publishing Inc., 1980.

Mendelsohn, Robert S., M.D. *Confessions of a Medical Heretic.* Contemporary Books, 1979.

Michaels, Joseph. *Prime of Your Life; a Practical Guide to Your Mature Years.* Little, Brown; 1981.

Montagu, Ashley. *Touching; the Human Significance of the Skin.* Columbia University Press, 1971.

Morris, Desmond. *The Human Zoo.* McGraw Hill, 1969.

National Academy of Sciences. *Diet, Nutrition and Cancer.* National Academy Press, 1982.

Notelovitz, Morris, Ph.D., M.D. *Stand Tall; the Informed Woman's Guide to Preventing Osteoporosis.* Gainesville, Florida; Triad Publishing, 1982.

Ormish, Dean, M.D. *Stress, Diet and Your Heart.* Holt, Rhinehart and Winston, 1982.

Pauling, Linus; Cameron, Ewing. *Cancer and Vitamin C.* Menlo Park, California; Linus Pauling Institute, 1975.

Pelletier, Kenneth L., Ph.D. *Mind as Healer, Mind as Slayer.* Delta Books, 1977.

_____ *Holistic Medicine; from Stress to Optimum Health.* Delacorte, 1979.

_____ *Longevity: Fulfilling Our Biological Heritage.* Delacorte, 1981.

Pitskhelauri, G.Z., M.D. *The Long Living of Soviet Georgia.* Soviet Academy Press, 1978.

Pritikin, Nathan; McGrady, P.M. *The Pritikin Program for Diet and Exercise.* Grosset and Dunlap, 1979.

Reisberg, Barry. *Brain Failure; an Introduction to the Current Concept of Senility.* The Free Press, 1981.

Robinson, Vera, M.D. *Humor and the Health Profession.* Slack Press, 1977.

Rosenfeld, Albert. *Pro-Longevity.* Aron Books, 1977.

Segersberg, Osborn, Jr. *Living to Be 100.* Charles Scribner and Sons, 1982.

Serfass, Robert; Smith, Everett L. *Exercise and Aging.* Enslow Publishers, 1981.

Silverstein, Alvin. *Conquest of Death.* MacMillan, 1979.

Simonton O. Carl, M.D.; Simonton, Stephanie-Mathews; Creighton, J. *Getting Well Again.* J.P. Tarcher, 1978.

Smith, Lendon, M.D. *Feed Yourself Right.* McGraw Hill, 1983.

Starr, Paul. *The Social Transformation of American Medicine.* Basic Books, 1982.

Strehler, Bernard L., Ph.D. *Time, Cells and Aging.,* 2nd edition. Academy Press, 1977.

Sutphen, Dick and Trenna. *Master of Life Manual.* Scottsdale, Arizona; Valley of the Sun Publishing, 1980.

Vaillant, George. *Adaption to Life; How the Best and Brightest Came of Age.* Little, Brown; 1977.

Wallace, Gordon. *The Valiant Heart; From Cardiac Cripple to World Champion.* Prescott, Arizona; Ralph Tauser Associates, 1981.

Walford, Roy L., Ph.D. *Maximum Life Span.* W. W. Norton, 1983.

Walton, Lewis R.; Walton, Jo Ellen; Scharffenburg, John A., M.D. *How You Can Live Six Extra Years.* Woodbridge Press, 1981.

Willing, Jules Z. *The Lively Mind.* William Morrow, 1982.

Woodruff, Diana S., Ph.D. *Can You Live to Be 100?* Chatham Square Press, 1977.

Periodicals and Pamphlets

American Association of Retired Persons. *Your Retirement Health Guide.* AARP Press, 1977.

Bauer, Lee. Editor, writing in various issues of *Your Health* Newsletter. Kailua, Hawaii, 1982–3.

Berkman, Lisa F., Ph.D. "Study on Social Bonds." *American Journal of Epidemiology,* February 1979.

Breakey, Jeff. Editor, writing in various issues of *The Sproutletter.* Ashland, Oregon; 1982–3.

Breiner, S. J. "Causes of Death—Unconsciousness Dimensions." *Current Concepts in Psychology;* March-April 1978, pp 17–22.

Brill, P. "Work Satisfaction Best Predictor of Longevity." *American Medical News;* December 1, 1978; p 16.

Brody, Jane E. "Marriage Is Good for Health and Longevity, Studies Say." *New York Times (Science Times);* May 8, 1979, pp 1–2.

Castelli, William P., M.D. "Summary Estimates of Cholesterol Used to Predict Coronary Heart Disease." *Circulation*; Vol 67, No. 4, April 1983.

Committee for an Extended Lifespan. *Immortality* and *Lifelines Newsletters*. CFEL, 1971–1981.

Drori, D., M.D.; Folman, Y., M.D. "Environmental Effect on Longevity in the Male Rat." *Experimental Gerontology*; II, 1976, pp 25–32.

Greenberg L.J.; Yunis, E.J. "Histocompatibility Determinants, Immune Responsiveness, and Aging in Man." *Federal Proceedings*; April, 1978, 37(5), pp 1258–1262.

Hall, Howard R. "Hypnosis and the Immune System; a Review with Implications for Cancer and the Psychology of Healing." *American Journal of Clinical Hypnosis*; Vol 25, #2–3, October 1982-January 1983.

Hepner, G.; Fried, R.; Jeor, S.S. "Hypercholesterolemic Effect of Yogurt and Milk." *American Journal of Clinical Nutrition*; 1979, pp 19–24.

International Federation on Aging. *Aging International* Newsletter, various issues.

Jewette, S. P. "Longevity and the Longevity Syndrome." *Gerontologist*; Spring 1973, pp 91–99.

Kallman, F. J.; Sander, G. "Twin Studies on Senescence." *American Journal of Psychiatry*; 1949, 106, 29.

Karasek, Robert, Ph.D. "Jobs Where Stress is Most Severe." *U.S. News*; September 5, 1983, pp 45.

Lachance, P.A. "The Role of Cereal Grain Products in the U.S. Diet." *Food Technology*; March 1981, pp 49–60.

Leon, A.S.; Blackburn, H. "The Relationship of Physical Activity to Coronary Heart Disease and Life Expectancy." *Annals of the New York Academy of Sciences*; 1977, pp 561–578.

Palmore, Erdman B. Ph.D. "Physical, Mental and Social Factors in Predicting Longevity." *Gerontologist*; Summer, 1969. pp 103–108.

Ponce de Leon Letter, various issues. Life Extension Center of Warren Research, Decatur, Illinois.

Report: "Looking for the Fountain of Youth." *Science Digest*; July 1983, pp 90.

Sauer, H.I., M.D.; Parke, D.W., M.D. "Counties with Extreme Death Rates and Associated Factors." *American Journal of Epidemiology*; 1979, 99, pp 258–264.

Science and Technology Department: "The Unsolved Riddle of Why People Age." *The Economist*; January 10, 1981.

Social Security Administration. *America's Centenarians*. Fourteen-volume series of interviews.

Troll, Walter, Ph.D. "Adding Seeds to the Diet May Keep Cancer at Bay," *Journal of the AMA;* May 27, 1983.

Vaughn, Lewis. "Life Extension; a Practical Guide." *Prevention;* April, 1983.

Vaux, Kenneth. "Religion and Health." *Preventative Medicine;* December 1976, pp 522–536.

Waldron, Ingrid. "Why Do Women Live Longer Than Men?" *Journal of Human Stress;* March 1976, pp 2–13.

Whitaker, Julian M., M.D. "Four Steps for Artery Clean Up." *Let's Live,* July 1981.

Index

The following pages feature more fine health and lifestyle titles from

PARA RESEARCH, INC.

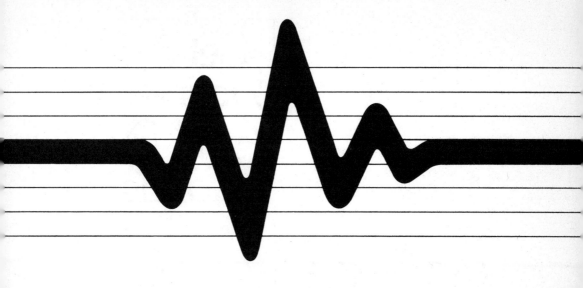

GOOD NIGHT

Norman Ford

Insomnia can be overcome naturally, without the use of drugs. *Good Night* is the book that tells you all about sleeping, insomnia and learning how to sleep again. Professional health writer Norman Ford has studied the insomnia problem and synthesized the work being done to fight it.

Recent studies indicate that almost 20 percent of Americans suffer from one or more of the six major forms of insomnia. This all too common problem is making us irritable and adding more stress to our already stressful world. Insomnia can be overcome by first understanding what it is that keeps us awake and then implementing the proper steps to help us sleep well again. After investigating the causes of sleeplessness, *Good Night* tells insomniacs what not to do and presents several programs which will assure the best possible night's sleep.

This is a comprehensive book that tells the reader how to achieve a healthier lifestyle through better sleep. This book will tell you what good sleep is, why drugs and medical techniques probably won't help you sleep and what you can do to sleep better naturally. *Good Night* is the one personal investment that is guaranteed to make you sleep better at night.

ISBN 0-914918-47-8
208 pages, 6½″×9¼″, paper $8.95

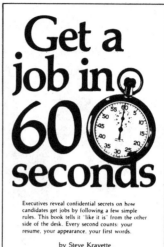

Get a job in 60 seconds

Executives reveal confidential secrets on how candidates get jobs by following a few simple rules. This book tells it "like it is" from the other side of the desk. Every second counts: your resume, your appearance, your first words.

by Steve Kravette

GET A JOB IN 60 SECONDS

Steve Kravette

First impressions. Those are what get you a job or cause you to lose it. According to Steve Kravette, the person doing the hiring looks at you and your application at certain critical points for five seconds and forms an opinion. If you hold the interviewer's attention for the full five seconds, you advance to the next stage of the process. If not, your resume goes into the wastebasket. Once all those five second segments add up to 60 seconds, you've got the job you want.

Kravette's new book is brisk, outspoken and loud. He talked to the people who make the real decisions about hiring in some of the largest companies in the country. Combining this with his own experience in getting jobs and hiring people, he crystallized this unique approach to the most important task facing people today.

Get A Job In 60 Seconds takes the job hunter through all the major stages of getting a job. It tells the applicants what their mind-set should be and how they can beat the odds to keep the interviewer's attention focused on them and off the other candidates.

Complete and yet concise, this book is different from other books in the market in its basic approach. Employment manuals ask you to do complicated and time consuming exercises. *Get A Job In 60 Seconds* is not a manual. It is a direct ticket to employment. It relays its message in a boiled down fashion that gets the 60 second technique across. And the basic premise is reinforced at the end of each chapter as you see how to gain important seconds through a variety of graphics.

ISBN 0-914918-41-9
144 pages, 5¼" x 8", paper $5.95

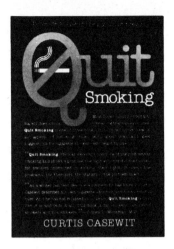

QUIT SMOKING

by Curtis Casewit

Author Curtis Casewit calls smoking the new social stigma. Never before has there been such a clear, concise and complete guide to the dangers of smoking and how to stop. *Quit Smoking* is sure to convince any smoker that he or she ought to stop, and best of all, it gives them the means.

Quit Smoking presents over 40 techniques which can help anyone stop smoking forever. Casewit surveys cessation programs all over the world to present as complete a guide on how to stop smoking as possible. Casewit's aim is twofold: first, he presents a number of individual stop smoking programs for the person who wants to stop on his or her own. Second, he reviews the major group cessation programs for those who need the support of others working to conquer the same problem.

From self-hypnosis to the Seventh Day Adventist Five Day Stop Smoking Plan, Casewit has done a truly major survey of the most successful methods used to stop smoking. *Quit Smoking* is full of charts on the effects of smoking and contains a detailed description of how the powerful tobacco lobby works for the interest of the cigarette industry in the United States.

Curtis Casewit is a former smoker and author of over 20 books. He began collecting information for this book when he quit his two pack a day habit. He was successful, and millions of other smokers can discover their own successful methods in *Quit Smoking*.

Introduction by Sidney L. Werkman, M.D.
ISBN 0-914918-44-3
144 pages, paper $7.95

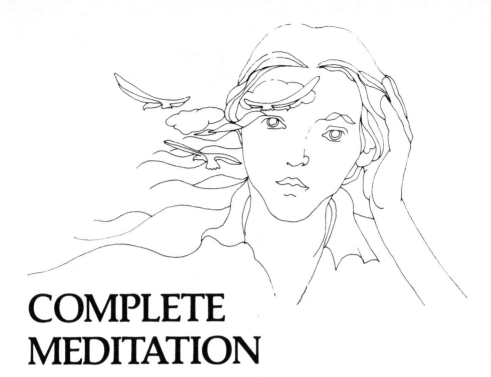

COMPLETE
MEDITATION

Steve Kravette

Complete Meditation presents a broad range of metaphysical concepts and meditation techniques in the same direct, easy-to-assimilate style of the author's best-selling *Complete Relaxation*. Personal experience is the teacher and this unique book is your guide. The free, poetic format leads you through a series of exercises that build on each other, starting with breathing patterns, visualization exercises and a growing confidence that meditation is easy and pleasurable. Graceful illustrations flow along with the text.

 Complete Meditation is for readers at all levels of experience. It makes advanced metaphysics and esoteric practices accessible without years of study of the literature, attachment to gurus or initiation into secret societies. Everyone can meditate, everyone is psychic, and with only a little attention everyone can bring oneself and one's circumstances into harmony.

 Experienced meditators will appreciate the more advanced techniques, including more sophisticated breathing patterns, astral travel, past-life regression, and much more. All readers will appreciate being shown how ordinarily "boring" experiences are really illuminating gateways into the complete meditation experience. Whether you do all the exercises or not, just reading this book is a pleasure.

 Complete meditation can happen anywhere, any time, in thousands of different ways. A candle flame, a daydream, music, sex, a glint of light on your ring. In virtually any circumstances. *Complete Meditation* shows you how.

ISBN 0-914918-28-1
309 pages, 6½" x 9¼", paper, $10.95

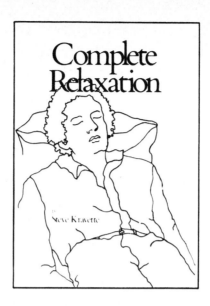

COMPLETE RELAXATION

Steve Kravette

Complete Relaxation is unique in its field because, unlike most relaxation books, it takes a completely relaxed approach to its subject. You will find a series of poetic explorations interspersed with text and beautifully drawn illustrations designed to put you in closer touch with yourself and the people around you. *Complete Relaxation* is written for all of you: your body, your mind, your emotions, your spirituality, your sexuality—the whole person you are and are meant to be.

As you read this book, you will begin to feel yourself entering a way of life more completely relaxed than you ever thought possible. Reviewer Ben Reuven stated in the *Los Angeles Times*, "*Complete Relaxation* came along at just the right time—I read it, tried it; it works."

Some of the many areas that the author touches upon are: becoming aware, instant relaxation, stretching, hatha yoga, Arica, bioenergetics, Tai chi, dancing, and the Relaxation Reflex.

Mantras, meditating, emotional relaxation, holding back and letting go, learning to accept yourself, business relaxation, driving relaxation.

Family relaxation, nutritional relaxation, spiritual relaxation, sensual relaxation, massage and sexual relaxation. *Complete Relaxation* is a book the world has been tensely, nervously, anxiously waiting for. Here it is. Read it and relax.

ISBN 0-914918-14-1
310 pages, 6½" x 9¼", paper

$10.95

Norman Ford

Norman Ford is a medical researcher and self-help author, as well as an expert in holistic therapies. He has written for *Prevention* and *Bestways* as well as other popular health publications. He is the author of more than 40 books in the fields of travel, leisure and health, including: *Good Night, Good Health Without Drugs, Secrets of Staying Young and Living Longer, Natural Ways to Relieve Pain* and *Minding Your Body.* Mr. Ford lives in Boulder, Colorado, and is an avid outdoorsman, hiker, bicyclist, swimmer and jogger.